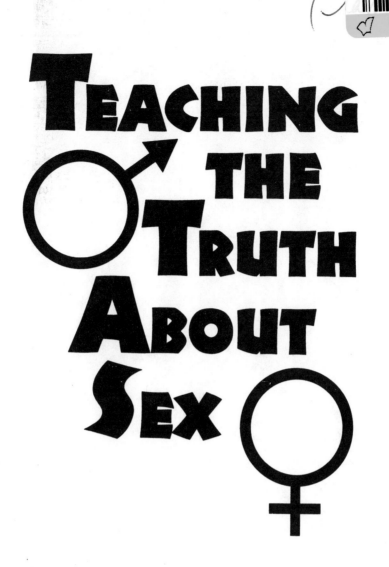

Teaching the Truth About Sex

Other Zondervan/Youth Specialties Books

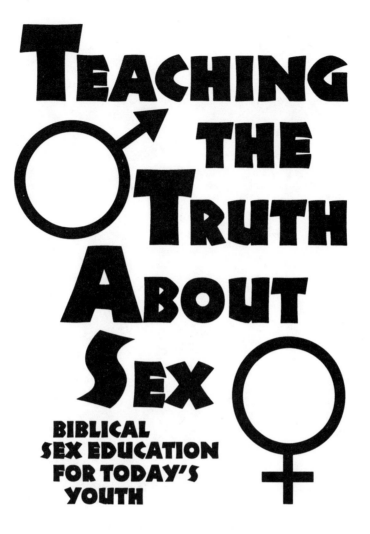

TEACHING THE TRUTH ABOUT SEX

BIBLICAL SEX EDUCATION FOR TODAY'S YOUTH

DAVID LYNN *and* MIKE YACONELLI

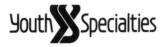

Youth Specialties

Zondervan Publishing House
Grand Rapids, Michigan

Teaching the Truth About Sex

Copyright © 1990 by Youth Specialties, Inc.

Youth Specialties Books, 1224 Greenfield Drive, El Cajon, California 92021,
are published by Zondervan Publishing House,
1415 Lake Drive, S.E., Grand Rapids, Michigan 49506

Library of Congress Cataloging in Publication Data

Lynn, David, 1954–
    Teaching the truth about sex : biblical sex education for today's youth / by
David Lynn and Mike Yaconelli.
      p.   cm.
    ISBN 0-310-52531-4
    1. Sex—Religious aspects—Christianity. 2. Sex instruction for teenagers. I.
Yaconelli, Mike. II. Title.
BT708.L96 1990
241'.66—dc20   89-48029
                                                   CIP

All Scripture quotations, unless otherwise noted, are taken from the *Holy Bible:
New International Version* (North American Edition). Copyright © 1973, 1978,
1984, by the International Bible Society. Used by permission of Zondervan Bible
Publishers.

Designed by Jack Rogers
Typeset by Leah Perry

Printed in the United States of America

90 91 92 93 94 95 / DP / 12 11 10 9 8 7 6 5 4 3 2

TABLE OF CONTENTS

INTRODUCTION AND PHILOSOPHY

- A five-year-old says to his friend, "I found a condom on the patio." His friend asks, "What's a patio?"
- A college-age couple visits their youth worker. The girl is pregnant, they're not married, and both are very upset. They're not upset *because* she's pregnant—they can't understand *why* she's pregnant. They asked God to keep her from getting pregnant every time they had sex.
- A study compared the sexual behavior of high school young people with no church affiliation with high school young people who attend church regularly. There was no difference.
- Told that their high school daughter was sexually promiscuous, parents replied, "Frankly, we'd rather not know because we don't want to deal with it."

It's about time! It's about time someone developed a curriculum about sex that *realistically* deals with the sexual pressures facing the young people in high school today. When five-year-olds know more about condoms than patios, when adolescents ask God to condone sexual intercourse before marriage, when the Christian faith makes no difference in adolescent sexual behavior, when parents don't want to get involved, then those of us who work with adolescents have to find a way to *realistically* confront today's sexual relativity with biblical values. This curriculum is an effective answer to that dilemma.

We emphasize the word *"realistically"* because we believe that for any curriculum to be effective with adolescents, it has to reflect where kids are today, not where they were five years ago. To that end, we have based our approach on five assumptions.

1. Most of today's sex education is ineffective and counterproductive. There. We've said it and we're glad. Too many people are afraid to admit that "values neutral" education, in fact, teaches all the wrong values (sex is just a physical act, sexual behavior has no consequences, sex is a "technical" skill rather than a moral act, and so on). Today's sex education gives young people knowledge they don't know what to do with. It's like "educating" ten-year-olds on how to make a time bomb and giving them the materials without discussing the moral implications of blowing up human beings.

The authors believe that modern sex education *increases* the sexual pressure on adolescents. They learn *what* to do but not how to decide when, where, with whom, and under what circumstances. Those are moral questions and adolescents need help learning how to answer them. This curriculum provides that help.

2. The majority of churches are not talking about sex. The liberal church has adopted the values-neutral approach to sex education. The conservative church has long held

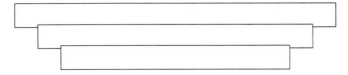

that the less adolescents know about sex, the less likely they are to engage in sexual activity. We have sympathy with that point of view, but there is one major problem. *Our kids are getting a sex education.* Silence does not protect young people. It only makes them more vulnerable to the sources of modern sex "education"—MTV, movies, peers, magazines, and television.

3. Many parents are not talking with their children about sex. Most parents assume their children know their sexual ethics and would rather not sit down face-to-face and go through the unpleasant awkwardness of talking about sex. So they leave sex education to others.

4. Sex education is more complex than it was a few years ago. Just a few years ago, adolescents didn't know anything about oral sex, vibrators, sado-masochism, sodomy, orgasms, anal sex, incest, lesbianism, and homosexuality. They do now.

5. Sexual contact has accelerated among adolescents. Our young people have more sexual involvement with more partners at a younger age than previous generations.

• It is not unusual for children from sixth grade up to experience heavy kissing and sexual touching on the first date. Kissing, even French kissing, has lost its meaning and is done indiscriminately. Sexual intimacy is becoming a substitute for normal relations with family and friends. Living together is commonly viewed as a prerequisite to marriage.

• The double standard is disappearing. Young women are still judged more harshly than young men for casual sexual activity, but they are no longer looked down upon if they sleep with their boyfriends.

• Masturbation has been legitimized. Always popular among males, masturbation is increasingly practiced among females. The consequences of its popularity with both sexes are serious—increased sexual fantasy, more emphasis on sex as a physical experience, selfish sex, orgasm viewed as the only object of sex, and so on.

• The incidence of sexually transmitted diseases (STDs) is on the increase among adolescents. Young people believe they are basically immune from STDs or AIDS. Since they are just beginning their sexual contacts, they think they don't need to fear diseases transmitted by older people who have had many sexual partners.

• Birth control is more available. In addition to the ever-present condoms, many girls can get birth control pills easily and without parental permission.

It's painfully clear that today's adolescents are the real casualties of the sexual revolution of the sixties. They have been catapulted into a moral vacuum created by the previous generation, totally unprepared for the sexual pressures they face. Whether we want to admit it or not, the influence of the Christian faith has been successfully removed from the modern sexual ethic so that sexuality is thoroughly secularized. What this means is that the church's response to the adolescent sexual crisis is more critical than ever!

But Should the Church Be Talking About Sex?

Yes! Talking frankly about sex does not violate its sacredness. Many churches, if they have talked about sex at all, have avoided discussing the specifics of sexual behavior because they feared diminishing the sacredness of sex. That may have been the case when adolescents had limited sexual knowledge, but it isn't the case any longer. The church must restore the sacredness of sex by discussing it in the context of a biblical value system. Obviously, some sexual terms are inappropriate, but the technical

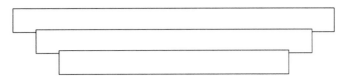

terms for sexual behavior should be used.

Sex education in the church means not only teaching young people to say no to sex, but providing things for them to say yes to. Simply asking kids to repress their sexual urges only leads them into sexual sin. We need to give them permission to be sexual beings in ways that are pleasing to God.

Sex education in the church does not encourage or condone sexual behavior. Quite the contrary, it is the only place where young people will be exposed to a biblical perspective about sex. Not just a technical explanation, it is a discussion of the implications of biblical truth on all of life, from the worth of the individual, to the meaning of love and commitment, to the cost of discipleship.

Don't We Need to Begin With a Philosophy?

Indeed we do, and we have a choice. Two basic philosophies have dominated sex education over the last twenty years. The first, "moral certainties," teaches that moral absolutes need to be known, understood, and respected if one is to have an adequate sex education. A moral certainties approach educates young people about sex and offers a moral code that influences all life decisions, including sex.

The second philosophy, "normative consequences," is probably the dominant approach in sex education courses today. It's based on the premise that right and wrong are determined by consequence. Therefore, a particular behavior, such as sexual intercourse, is normative (neither right nor wrong). If a couple has sexual intercourse and one person develops AIDS or a STD, sexual intercourse was not morally wrong—it was irresponsible. Responsible decision making is the focus of this philosophy. It teaches that the purpose of sex education is to equip young people with the information they need, if they are sexually active, to avoid unwanted pregnancies and STDs.

The AIDS epidemic has heightened the sex education controversy. Those who believe in moral certainties have increased their call for sexual abstinence until marriage. They accuse those who believe in "responsible" sex of encouraging the irresponsible sexual activity that has increased the incidence of unwanted pregnancy, abortion, and STDs.

Those who believe in normative consequences accuse the moral certainties group of being unrealistic. They contend that you can't stop adolescent sexual activity. In fact, they say, by telling adolescents that all sexual activity is wrong and refusing to differentiate between responsible and irresponsible sex, we send adolescents into a sexual reality without any defense. They believe it is inevitable that teenagers will be sexually active; therefore, it is unconscionable not to provide them with information regarding contraception, safe sex practices, and abortion.

So Which Philosophy Does This Curriculum Follow?

Because the consensus in this society is that abstinence is an unrealistic dream for most adolescents, the normative consequences approach to sex education has broad support, even among church programs.

Nevertheless, these authors reject this philosophy. We do not believe that sexual activity is inevitable for adolescents, although we concede that, given the current sexual climate, sexual abstinence is difficult.

That leaves us with the moral certainties approach. We feel it is theologically sound, but educationally ineffective. It's true to the biblical ideal, but insensitive to the human reality. Let's look at some of its weaknesses:
- *It's too simplistic.* The moral certainties

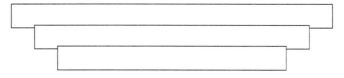

philosophy encourages adolescents to "just say no." But does telling young people to say "no" change behavior? Telling boys to keep their zippers up and girls to keep their legs crossed sounds very reassuring to adults, but the sexual pressure cooker that adolescents live in makes that difficult. It's easy to say "no" to sex in Sunday school, but much more difficult in a world that encourages everyone to say "yes." Young people need to do more than *say* "no"—they must understand *why*. Saying "no" must be a response to a conviction based on a belief system.

• *The church often preaches sex education instead of teaching it.* Sex education is most effective when it is taught instead of preached. Teaching implies interaction, with the student not only listening but understanding and experiencing. The common assumption is that if young people hear the truth, they will live it. Logic, experience, and Scripture tell us otherwise. Knowing is not doing. James tells us we must be more than hearers of the word (James 1:22-25). Adolescents can listen to someone talk about sexuality and agree with what they say, but that does not mean they will change their sexual behavior.

• *The church has emphasized what to do instead of teaching adolescents how to decide what to do.* The church often absolutizes the particulars of sexual behavior (don't kiss on the first date) without teaching the absolutes (our bodies are the temple of God). The church should provide biblical guidance and principles from Scripture, but the decisions must be left up to the adolescents. Christianity provides a foundation upon which we can make sound decisions on the particulars of life.

So how do we counteract these weaknesses in our chosen approach? By:

• *Listening to kids.* Let the young people talk openly about the real pressures they are under.

• *Asking them what they need to know.* Often sex education assumes the kids want to know biology when they really want to know how to control the biological urges they have.

• *Talking about sex frankly.* Saying "no" to sex means what? You hold hands until you get married? Adolescents want to know if they also need to say "no" to masturbation, oral sex, and heavy kissing for five hours.

• *Not assuming the young people know what you are talking about.* In spite of today's sex education, many adolescents are ignorant and naive when it comes to sex.

• *Not assuming that "the Bible says" or "God is against" has any effect.* Sadly, the Bible and God do not carry much weight with many adolescents, even those in the church. Obviously, it is important to know what the Bible and God say about sexual behavior, but we shouldn't be surprised if it doesn't have much impact.

• *Talking about consequences.* Just because the "normative consequence" people talk about consequences doesn't mean we can't. Adolescents need to know that the Bible doesn't arbitrarily say things are wrong. It says they are wrong for a reason.

This is a skills-based curriculum founded on a *realistic* moral certainties approach. The authors are committed to the absolutes of the Gospel *and* the skills required to live out the implications of those absolutes. Young people need more from sex education than information; they need the skills to make sexual decisions that are consistent with biblical truth. This material will help make that goal a reality.

LEADER'S GUIDE

Getting Acquainted with the Sessions

Each session offers the following sections, but you will choose those that meet the needs of your group:

Session Purpose

This concise statement allows you as a leader to focus on the specific subject matter to be covered and the goals of the exercises. You may decide to extend or narrow the focus. Or you can emphasize one aspect of the subject if that is appropriate for your group.

Background Brief

This section helps the leader see the context of the problem so the discussion will not be held in a vacuum. What are the issues for adolescents? What biblical and spiritual dilemmas are involved? What are the areas of conflict and how can they be resolved? For example, one Background Brief will warn you that adolescents today assume premarital sex is okay if you love your partner. So in your discussion you not only have to talk about *what* is right, but how to *do* what is right when everyone says you are wrong.

After the Background Brief comes the session itself, which includes at least several if not all of the following exercises:

Group Starters. This exercise enables young people to focus their attention on the topic of the session.

Thinking Starters. Discussion questions and activities ask young people to think about the implications of the issue in their own lives.

Discussion Starters. The young people listen to other viewpoints and decide whether to defend their own belief, abandon it in favor of another point of view, or alter it.

Faith Starters. The focus changes to what God has to say about the issue. Relevant Scripture encourages discussion of the spiritual and biblical dimensions of the issue.

Action Starters. Through these activities young people act on what they have learned. They are challenged to live out their belief in the real world.

Reflection Starters. At the end of the session the young people consider and analyze what they have learned.

Parent Discussion Guide

This handout lets the families know what you have discussed and encourages them to continue the discussion at home.

Preparing for a Session

• **Read the entire session.** Note the exercises that you think will work best with your group and, if you wish, alter them in any way you think is appropriate. Be selective and use *only* the material you think will work with your group within your time constraints. We've included far too much for most sessions, so choose what is valuable for you.

Use the handouts as handouts—or add variety to the session by copying the information on a large chart, making it into an overhead, or even reading it aloud. If you know a resource that would fit into a particular session or you want to add your own material, feel free to do so.

• **Try to write in one sentence your goal for this session.** It may be different from the one printed in the material. You are the best qualified to decide where you want this session to go.

• **Decide whether you will need help with the session.** Depending on your own knowledge of Scripture, you may want to ask the pastor or minister of your church to help with—or even conduct—some of the sessions. This person could help explain your denomination's beliefs concerning sensitive topics, such as homosexuality.

• **Use a particular session whenever you want, in whatever order you want.** Don't feel you have to offer every session or offer them in order. They're designed to be flexible!

Facilitating Effective Discussions

• **Create an atmosphere of openness and acceptance.** Adolescents must feel free to express their opinions without being condemned, criticized, or ostracized. This does not mean that you tolerate crude or inappropriate comments, but do allow young people to say what they really believe, whether you or the rest of the class agree with them or not. Openness lets young people work out their opinions in a community of people who will listen without judging them.

One way to create a climate of acceptance is to encourage *opinions*, not *answers*. Instead of asking "What is wrong with masturbation?" ask "What do you think about masturbation?" The phrase "what do you think" makes it easier for adolescents to give their opinions without worrying whether they have the right answer.

At the same time, be careful that your openness is not misinterpreted as permission to sin. Don't let the effort to maintain openness keep you from confronting adolescents when they state opinions that contradict what the Bible teaches about sex. You want kids to share what they believe without fear of rejection, but you can still disagree with what they are saying. (Obviously, in rare cases where someone is attempting to dominate or shock the group, you may have to step in and cut the person off. But after the meeting try to talk with him or her privately about what happened.)

• **Maintain strict confidentiality.** Discuss the need for this at your first session. For young people to be open and honest, they have to trust that what they say will not be repeated outside the session by you or anyone else in the group. They have to trust that when they open up, you won't make a public example out of them, reject them, think less of them, or criticize them. Assume conversations or statements are confidential unless otherwise stated. Don't use experiences shared in the group or in private as illustrations (even

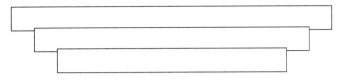

when disguised) unless you have permission.

On the other hand, don't let confidentiality hold you to secrecy no matter what. Carefully define the exceptions to confidentiality at the beginning of the course. Tell the young people that sometimes confidentiality must be broken so you can help them, particularly when the situation is life threatening or sexual or physical abuse is involved. (This is mandated by law in many states.)

In many situations you are obligated to keep the information confidential, but you can still encourage the adolescent to tell a parent or someone else who can help. (If a girl was date raped, for example.) Offer to go with the young person.

If you do feel it necessary to break a confidence, say as little as necessary to as few people as necessary. Tell only those who must know, only those who can directly help the adolescent and his or her family.

• **Be careful about public confessions.** In recent years some pregnant girls have confessed their sin to their youth groups. The groups have helped the girls through their pregnancies, even going into the delivery room. Experiences like these can be positive in the short term, but negative in the long term. In the beginning, the youth group feels supportive and helpful, and the pregnant girl feels loved and accepted. But after the birth, the girl may be forgotten and long for the attention she received when she was pregnant. Before you encourage this type of confession, thoroughly discuss how to handle the situation with experienced adults and counselors.

• **Encourage young people to contribute, even when you don't agree with their opinions.** Periodically make statements

such as these:

"That's a good point, Bob."
"Interesting idea, Linda. Not too many of us have thought about that."
"Good question, Carrie."
"Obviously, Daryl has given this a lot of thought."
"Diana has some strong feelings about this subject. That took a lot of courage."

You will not comment every time someone shares, of course, but affirming young people's contributions is an effective way to stimulate participation and build trust between you and your class.

• **Encourage discussions without becoming the center of them.** Allow young people to discuss the issues with each other and avoid taking sides during the disagreements. Instead, encourage both sides to think through their positions and defend their points of view. If everyone seems to agree or if people seem reluctant to express a controversial viewpoint, you might want to play the devil's advocate and, for the sake of the discussion, raise another point of view and defend it. Preface your remarks by saying something like, "What about people who say . . ." The best discussion leader is one who can remain neutral. Nevertheless, you can and should give your point of view at the end of the session during your concluding remarks.

• **Stimulate participation when people seem hesitant to talk.** Pass out cards and have young people write down their thoughts on a subject anonymously. Collect the cards, read them aloud, and ask the group to respond.

Take a test or a survey. Then go over the questions and have the young people

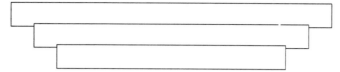

respond to each one. Or have them turn in their tests or surveys and read aloud the written responses without identifying the writers.

Videotape an interview with volunteer young people and show it to the group. (Obviously, make sure the volunteers know the video will be shown.)

Record part of a movie or MTV video, play it for the group, and discuss it.

Have everyone read copies of a magazine article dealing with the subject you are discussing and discuss it.

• **Allow some issues to remain unresolved.** Often an issue will not be resolvable, but exploring it is still valuable for the young people. Listening to others' opinions—and Scripture—helps young people shape their own viewpoints, even if the session ends with no consensus.

• **Don't feel you have to know all the answers.** Always feel free to ask knowledgeable people, such as your pastor or minister, to sit in on a discussion when you anticipate needing help. If you are conducting a session by yourself and discover you're not sure of your church's stand on a particular issue, invite your pastor or minister to attend the next session and help clarify it. Or ask one or more young people to interview an appropriate person concerning an issue and report their findings to the class. Young people will respect you for admitting you still have things to learn.

• **Stop the discussion when appropriate.** Stop if someone is getting upset, attacking another student, getting too intimate, or being disrespectful or crude. You could say:

"Okay, Bob, I think we have the jist of what you are saying. Let's move on now to another question."

"Let's try to keep our remarks from getting too personal."

"We have some very strong feelings being expressed right now. Why don't we take a break for a minute?"

Also stop the discussion if it's getting too long, one person is dominating the conversation, or it's not going anywhere. It's always better to end a discussion before everyone wants to rather than after everyone is bored.

Recognizing the Risks of Teaching Sex Education

Like most things worth doing, teaching sex education involves some risks. The main ones are overdoing it, becoming *too* involved with young people, and teaching half the truth.

Overdoing It

Often we assume that adolescents have discussed sexual issues in school and with their friends. The truth is that many adolescents are not sophisticated about sexual issues. They either have not paid attention in their sex education classes, or they are embarrassed about sex, or their parents have deliberately protected them from frank and open sexual discussion. Whatever the reason, teachers of sex education must be sensitive to their young people's receptivity. Here are some practical steps you can take to ensure you are not embarrassing or over-educating your young people:

• **If possible, meet with parents ahead of time.** Try to get their perception of their children's sexual sophistication. This way you can also find out what level of directness the parents are comfortable with.

• **Recognize that perhaps not all of your**

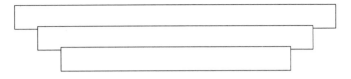

young people should participate in sessions on sex. Some adolescents are too young and some are unwilling to discuss such a sensitive area. The material is valuable for each student, but don't ask for total participation. Give young people an opportunity to "opt out" without losing face.

• **Don't assume the young people know what you are talking about.** Explain terms like "masturbation" and "oral sex" even if no one asks what they mean. Many kids won't admit what they don't know. Use only the words and terms that are necessary. Don't try to impress kids with the slang words you know.

• **Watch the group carefully.** If you notice they are getting quiet or certain kids are embarrassed, change the discussion to a more comfortable direction. After the meeting, *if it feels comfortable*, approach those you thought might be having a problem and tactfully probe to see if you were reading the situation correctly.

Becoming Too Involved With Young People

Tragically, there is an epidemic of sexual sin and youth ministers are not immune. To guard against the wrong kind of involvement with your young people:

• **Don't consider yourself immune to sexual temptation.** The fact that you are married, much older than your young people, an adult, or a minister is no guarantee that you won't end up in serious trouble. Discourage counseling sessions with a young person of the opposite sex. Avoid placing yourself in sexually tempting situations, such as flirting, wrestling, or spending hours alone with someone of the opposite sex. Young people in sexual crisis are extremely vulnerable.

• **Be sensitive to the issue of touching.** True, many young people need touch more than ever, but touch can be misunderstood. The media attention given to molestation and sexual abuse has been important in uncovering sexual sin, but the backlash has been a "molest mania" where even innocent touching is considered potential molestation. Today a youth worker cannot display physical affection without risk.

• **Stay in touch with your own sexuality.** If you and your spouse are having sexual difficulty, if you are a sensual person, if you are under stress or feeling lonely, you are in a potentially dangerous situation. Let someone else teach the course for a while and confide in an adult.

• **Maintain adult relationships.** The stronger your relationships with other adults, the less chance you have of making a mistake with young people.

• **Deal with inappropriate sexual behavior of other leaders directly and quickly.** If you are concerned about the behavior of another leader, get advice from a leader in the church and then confront the person involved. You do not have to be accusatory or judgmental, just concerned. The person may not even be aware he or she is creating a problem. Don't let fear of being wrong keep you from dealing with inappropriateness.

Teaching Half the Truth

In talking about sex with young people, state *all* the truth with conviction. Sexual sin has serious social and physical consequences, but sin is forgivable. We are to avoid sin, but God loves us even when we don't. Remember these two points:

1. Stress the intent of the law more than

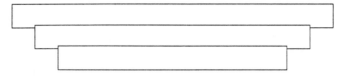

the law itself. God's sexual laws are to *protect* sex, not outlaw it. His principles of sexual behavior are meant to ensure that sexual experience within marriage is beautiful and positive.

2. Teach with compassion. Someone in your class probably has broken every sexual moral law you are discussing. You can still point out sexual sin and hold up the ideal, but you must teach the grace and forgiveness of God concurrently. For example, someone in your class may have had an abortion. It's too late *not* to have an abortion. Remind them—and the class—that God forgives.

Including Parents in the Program

This material is a resource for parents as well as adolescents. To include parents in the program:

Explain the curriculum to them and ask for their input. Invite parents to a meeting to discuss the curriculum. Hold it in another parent's home, not the church, and have the invitation come from a parent. (A sample letter is included in the Leader's Guide.) Let them see the curriculum material and explain to them how you will present it. Stress your policy of confidentiality and your biblical understanding of the issues. Ask for parents' suggestions and implement them whenever possible.

Also, send a letter home describing the material you presented in the parent meeting, for those parents who were hesitant or unable to come.

Send home the parent discussion sheets. Copy the sheet for each session, give one to each student attending, and suggest they use the sheets to continue your discussion at home.

Sponsor a meeting for parents called "How to Talk to Your Adolescent About Sex." A great deal of material is available on discussing sex with children, but here are a few of our suggestions to pass on to parents:

• Explain your own sexual values. Most adolescents know the technical information about sex, but they really don't know their parents' sexual values. Keep your comments short and avoid giving a lecture. At the same time, don't share your bedroom secrets. Sometimes parents reveal sexual intimacies to show their child how "cool" they are. This tends to confirm the idea that sex is just a physical act instead of a sacred secret between two people.

• Don't interpret lack of participation from your child as lack of interest. He or she is listening, but just too embarrassed to discuss the details. That's okay. Children still need to hear what their parents believe.

• Encourage your child to ask questions. (You don't have to answer any you feel are too intimate or those you simply don't know the answer to.) Try to maintain an attitude of openness. Admit to your own embarrassment and difficulty with discussing sex.

• If your child shares some upsetting glimpses of sexual attitude or behavior, don't punish him or her for being honest. Continue discussing the areas of concern, but don't impose emergency rules or limitations as the result of your conversation. Let's suppose, for example, that you discover your son is having sex with his girlfriend or your daughter is using birth control. Let them know that you are not in favor of such behavior and need to discuss how to resolve this issue. As a parent, you cannot condone what they're doing or look the other way. Be firm, loving, and supportive of them, not of what they are doing.

• Don't give ultimatums unless you are

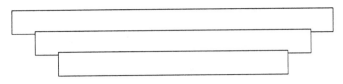

prepared to enforce them. And don't take responsibility for the consequences of their decisions. Explain what the consequences will be and help them understand that if they violate your expectations (which, hopefully, have been quietly and firmly communicated), they will have to live with the consequences *they* have chosen.

PARENT LETTER

January 1, 1990
Mr. and Mrs. Bob Smith
1469 Northstart Ave.
Tuscon, AZ 85704

Dear Bob and Mary,

   We'd like to invite you to a meeting in our home to discuss the series on sex that our youth director, Sandy Minton, is going to teach at the church. Harry and I have two children in the high-school group, Gary and Tim. Of course, we have a lot of confidence in Sandy, but, like any normal parent, we have some questions. We want to know exactly the areas Sandy is going to cover so we can support and benefit from these classes along with our children.

   So we have invited all the parents of the high-school group to attend a short session (an hour and a half) with Sandy to discuss the upcoming series. We would love for you to come. Please call us at 747-8654 and let us know if you're able to attend so we can have plenty of refreshments.

   We're enclosing a course outline that will give you a general idea of the topics covered. If you are unable to attend but have questions, please call Sandy at 748-2324.

                          Cordially,

                          Harry and Karla Connell

PARENT REFUSAL FORM

I do not want _____ to participate in the sexuality course.

(If you wish, please write us a note in the space below and let us know the reasons you would rather not have your child in the sexuality course.)

_____   _____
Parent's Signature   Date

SESSION ONE
SEX MAKES ME NERVOUS

Session Purposes

To establish an open and safe environment in which we can discuss sex and related issues. To help the young people explore their current sexual values. To begin our study of what the Bible says and doesn't say about sex. To determine what each person wants to learn from this series.

What creates openness and safety?

- *Honesty.* The more honest you are, the more open the young people will be.
- *Compassion.* If young people feel they can admit to failure without being judged, they will be more willing to share their thoughts and lives.
- *Protection.* Young people need to know they will be protected against ridicule and criticism when they share. Part of your job as a leader is to defend young people from other young people.
- *Empathy.* When young people realize that you understand, that you are a friend, that you remember what it's like to be an adolescent, they will open up to you.

Background Brief

Two false assumptions have been made about adolescent sex education: Secular sex education is adequate and parents and the church have communicated sexual values to adolescents.

In the Introduction we discussed the inadequacy of modern sex education. Concerning the second point, adolescents know the church and their parents still believe sexual intercourse should wait until marriage, but they don't really understand *why*. Nor do they understand what a Christian should do between holding hands and getting married. Either the church has told young people "Just say no" or, too often, it has refused to talk frankly and openly with adolescents about sex.

The material in this lesson enables your young people to talk, in a Christian environment, about the real issues they face sexually. They will also explore the implications of biblical truth and Christian faith for adolescent sexual behavior.

Group Starters

1. Introduce yourself and other leaders to the group. Let the young people know about your family, your background, your apprehensions, and your own struggles with sex when you were an adolescent. You don't need to tell the lurid details of your past, just that you struggled, too.

Optional: Pass out the "Was Our Leader a . . . SEX MANIAC?" sheet on page 23. Have the kids fill it out and then tell them the actual answers.

Tell them why you are excited about teaching this course and let them know from your heart how concerned you are for them. Explain that you know how rough it is to be an adolescent today and recognize the extreme pressures that adolescents face.

2. You have been provided with four Group Starter sheets ("Sexual Behavior" on page 24, "Your Body" on page 25, "Sexual Thoughts" on page 26, and "Sexual Values" on page 27). Choose the one(s) appropriate for your group and pass them out. Have the kids fill them out without putting their names on them. Explain that these sheets are provided to help you *and* them understand where they are sexually.

3. Write the word "Sex" on the board and ask the young people to brainstorm words and phrases they think of when they hear it. Write their responses (discouraging vulgar terms) on the board in a random pattern around the key word. After everyone has had an opportunity to suggest words, point out that sex means different things to all of us. In this course they are going to spend a lot of time talking and thinking about sex, finding out what they really believe, learning what the Bible says, and making some decisions about their own sex lives.

Stress that you want them to feel comfortable and to participate in discussions as much—or as little—as they want to. Emphasize that everything that is said in class is confidential. NOTHING can be repeated outside the classroom, to anyone, by anyone. In the same way, everything that is said in class will be

respected. No put-downs or insults are allowed.

Encourage the young people to share what they hope to learn from the course. Why did they decide to attend? What would they like to know? Is there anything they don't want to talk about in connection with sex?

Optional: During the preceding week ask some young people to videotape or audiotape people's responses to the word "sex." Play the tapes for the group and discuss them.

Thinking Starters

Have the kids each number a sheet of paper from 1 to 18. Read each item on the "I Believe" sheet on page 28 aloud and have them mark their papers "true" or "false."

Ask the young people to think for a minute about what they discovered in this exercise, without sharing their answers. Ask if anyone would like to share what they learned with the class.

Discussion Starters

Here are some options for using "Opinions" on page 29:
• Discuss each opinion with the class and try to come to a consensus as to how everyone feels about it. Encourage young people to try to convince the rest of the group their point of view is correct. Then vote as a group.
• Break into small groups (one adult in each group), discuss one of the opinions, and try to come to a consensus on the agree-disagree scale. Record the group's reasoning on the back of the opinion card. Then have the groups share their responses with the rest of the class.
• Or break into small groups and have each group take a different opinion card and try to reach consensus. Then come back together and ask each group to read

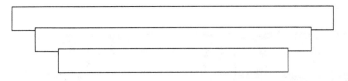

its situation and the response. The other groups can react.

• Duplicate the opinion cards and have the young people take them to school and ask others to write their response. At the next session, discuss the responses.

Faith Starters

Listed on the "Faith Starters" sheet on page 30 are Bible verses grouped under general topics. Divide the class into small groups, assign each group a category, and have them look up several of the Scriptures. Then ask each group to write a summary of what those Scriptures say regarding sex. At the end of the session, have each group write its summary on the board and explain it.

Action Starters

Pass out copies of the "Sex Attitudes Survey" on page 31 and ask the young people to have one or more of their friends respond to the questions anonymously. Explain that at the next session, you will compare what their friends think about the sexual issues included on the sheet.

Reflection Starters

Give everyone a copy of "Reflection Starters" on page 32 (or write one or more of the sentence stems on the board). Ask everyone to take a quiet moment to think about the session and complete the sentences, without writing their names on the paper. When everyone is finished, collect the papers. Stress that no one but you will read them, but you do want to know how they feel about this session and whether they have any suggestions for future sessions.

Take a few minutes to explain what you as a leader have learned during this session. Wrap up the meeting with some encouraging words from Scripture and ask a volunteer to close in prayer.

Session 1: Sex Makes Me Nervous

Teenagers today live in a different world than we did when we were their age. No one ever discussed AIDS with us, not many mentioned homosexuality, and only a few ever brought up the topic of sex.

The values in our society have changed dramatically over the last few years. We used to think that "good" boys and girls didn't get involved in sex, but in many ways those days are gone. In a recent survey by Josh McDowell of students who attend church regularly, 43% had intercourse by age 18, 35% of 17-year-olds said they have engaged in sexual intercourse, and 26% of 16-year-olds said they had had intercourse.

Further, our teens are bombarded with sexual messages. Everything from milk to wine coolers is marketed using sex appeal. It's easy to see how teens receive mixed signals concerning appropriate sexual behavior.

As one way to counteract these influences, try the discussion questions below with your son or daughter. Use them to build bridges of communication concerning sexuality. Be careful not to focus on the "right" answers; instead, listen to what your child thinks about the issues. Remember, communication is the key to having trust and dialogue with your young person.

Discussion Questions

For parents:
1. When did you start dating?

2. Did you have a lot of sexual pressure?

3. Did your faith influence your behavior back then?

4. What's the most important thing you think I should know about sex?

For the son or daughter:
1. Do you feel a lot of sexual pressure?

2. Is the course you're taking comfortable or uncomfortable?

3. Is it hard to talk to us about sexual matters? How could we make it easier?

4. What did you learn from this first lesson?

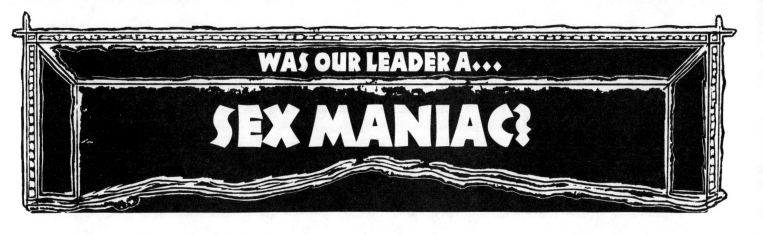

1. When our leader was a teenager:
   a. Sex hadn't been invented yet.
   b. Sex was a bad word.
   c. Holding hands was a big issue.
   d. Sex was discussed with words like "woo-woo" and "wee-wee."
   e. Couples actually dated.
   f. Sex was a major issue just like today.
   g. There wasn't as much sexual pressure.

2. Our leader's first romance occurred at the age of:
   a. 6 years old.
   b. Before twelve years old.
   c. Between 12 and 15.
   d. Between 16 and 19.
   e. After 20.
   f. 50.

3. The kind of kissing that was acceptable when our leader was in high school was:
   a. On the cheek.
   b. Open mouth.
   c. Open mouth—trade bubble gum.
   d. Snorkeler—come up periodically for air.
   e. Window fogger: hour-long marathons.
   f. None.

4. When our leader was in high school, the church basically believed:
   a. Sex is dirty . . . so save it until marriage.
   b. Sex is okay in marriage, but you can't enjoy it.
   c. Don't talk about sex.
   d. Sexual intercourse is only for marriage.
   e. Anything is okay as long as you don't do *it*.
   f. Whoopee!
   g. Mess around with sex and God will get you.

5. In high school our leader was considered:
   a. Stud.
   b. Fox.
   c. Macho.
   d. Prude.
   e. Prissy.
   f. Animal.
   g. Wimp.
   h. Loose.
   i. Clueless.
   j. Pre-pubescent.
   k. Wild lady.
   l. Fickle.
   m. Womanizer.
   n. Teaser.
   o. Sexy.
   p. Sensual.
   q. Respected.
   r. Moral.
   s. Flirt.
   t. Horny.
   u. Sensitive.
   v. Romeo.

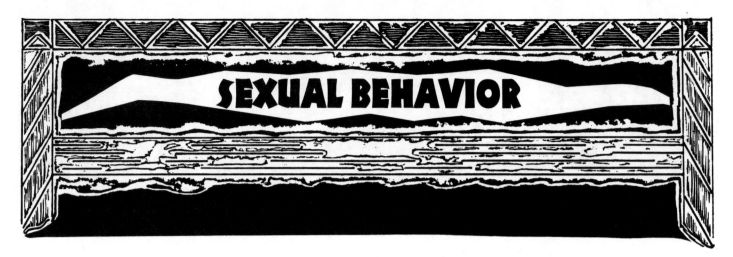

SEXUAL BEHAVIOR

Directions: Circle the words below that best describe how you feel about your sexual behavior (sexual conduct, masturbation, flirting, petting, etc.).

disgraceful	flaunting	perverted
guilty	godlike	smart
angry	defeated	sanctified
sorry	gratifying	careful
pure	discerning	respectful
forgiven	honorable	considerate
careless	virtuous	gamble
responsible	right	futile
godly	honest	cheap
injurious	good	unmarred
unhealthy	moral	spotless
spiritual	strict	fickle
sinful	tragic	proper
righteous	wrong	wicked
controlled	used	harmful
ethical	worthless	hurtful
biblical	immoral	depraved
ashamed	destructive	easy
embarrassed	helpless	flirty
innocent	scary	evil

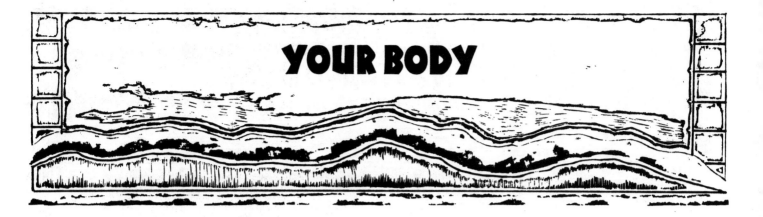

YOUR BODY

Directions: Circle the words below that best describe how you feel about your body (physical attractiveness, how you view your physical looks).

humorous	large	awesome
big	soft	worthless
healthy	husky	weak
foxy	dainty	cute
rejected	charming	sexy
thin	attractive	petite
hairy	energetic	sad
repulsive	masculine	feminine
wanted	gentle	fat
small	ugly	tall
strong	rare	flawed
pretty	skinny	perfect
tough	sensuous	useless
suffering	amusing	ordinary
well-built	well-dressed	pity
comfortable	changing	vain
homely	oversexed	sick
satisfactory	developed	deformed
deficient	disabled	childish
athletic	blemished	sissy
graceful	clumsy	short

SEXUAL THOUGHTS

Directions: Circle the words below that best describe how you feel about your sexual thoughts (sex, wishes, desires, etc.).

ungodly	strange	positive
disgusting	sick	explicit
wrong	weird	upright
innocent	divine	honorable
evil	abnormal	sorry
proper	holy	fabulous
exotic	disaster	unbelievable
gross	demented	good
spotless	help	arousing
perplexed	dangerous	forgiven
confused	great	futile
godlike	crazy	virtuous
helpless	sinful	angry
miserable	super	fantastic
pleasant	healthy	depraved
controlled	lustful	guilty
deprived	shameful	embarrassed
immoral	clean	destructive
rubbish	harmless	defeated
improving	scary	sanctified
	sensual	

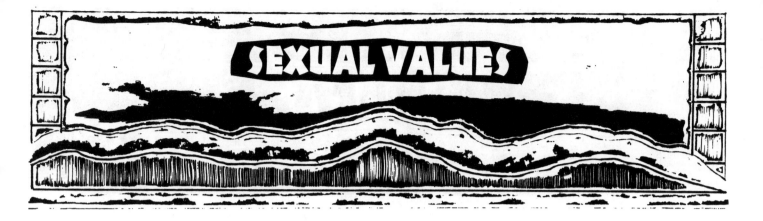

SEXUAL VALUES

Directions: Circle the words below that best describe how you feel about your sexual values (strongly held beliefs and attitudes).

unsettled	certain	strict
appropriate	puzzled	help
liberal	durable	godly
adequate	fickle	wholesome
questionable	fine	wise
pure	suitable	confused
secure	rigid	polluted
certain	open	set
disappointing	developed	growing
steadfast	clarified	deficient
changing	confused	ambiguous
proper	loose	reserved
improving	virtuous	childish
deteriorating	innocent	stable
endangered	established	inconsistent
flexible	uncertain	religious
acceptable	clear	moral
modest	biblical	spiritual
prudish	conservative	thought out
alarming	uncorrupted	inadequate
godly	wavering	responsible

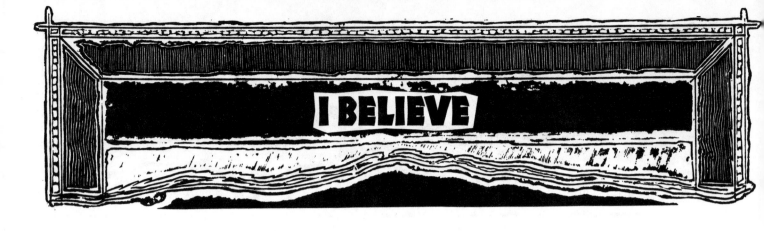

Instructions: Read some or all of these statements to your class and have them mark on sheets of paper "true" or "false."

1. The church's attitude towards sex is old fashioned.

2. My parents would be pleased with my sexual behavior.

3. Masturbation is normal for guys and girls.

4. A lot of kids never even have a date until college.

5. It's okay for couples to do anything sexually as long as they don't have intercourse.

6. God told people to wait until marriage to have sex for good reasons.

7. Television does not affect my sexual values.

8. I have no idea what the Bible says about sex.

9. Parents are impossible to talk to about sex.

10. Popular music has no effect on my sexual values.

11. I need to change my values and behaviors regarding sex.

12. A boy has the right to have sex if the girl has teased him.

13. My sex life is my own business.

14. I have lots of unanswered questions about sex.

15. I sometimes worry about homosexuality or lesbianism.

16. I believe in birth control.

17. I think abortion is wrong.

18. The best way to learn about sex is through experience.

CARRIE, 15-year-old sophomore. I had always been afraid of sex, but then I met this great guy. He's a senior and he's done it with other girls, so he knows what to do. What I mean is, he knew what to tell me to do and he made it much easier for me. He really does love me and for the first time in my life I can really say that I love him. And sex, contrary to what I've heard from my church and parents, is great. We don't do it every time we're together, but every time we do it, it's fantastic. How else can you show someone you love them?

☐ Agree ☐ Moderately Agree ☐ Moderately Disagree ☐ Disagree

LAUREN, 17-year-old junior. I'm a Christian and I really am trying to live like one. Sure, all the guys I go out with, including the Christian ones, keep pushing to have sex. But I'm not going to do it and if they don't like it, they can go with someone else. I think God had a reason for telling us to wait until marriage. Besides, the girls I know who are having sex with their boyfriends are always worried about breaking up or being pregnant. I have a couple of friends who ended up getting abortions and now they really are messed up. I'll admit I've wondered what it's like, but I'm not going to give in.

☐ Agree ☐ Moderately Agree ☐ Moderately Disagree ☐ Disagree

DON, 18-year-old senior. Look, I don't go out with girls I don't like. Obviously I like them or I wouldn't go out with them, so of course I expect to have sex. That's what a relationship is all about. You can't have a sort-of relationship. So, I mean, if after going out a few times, they don't care enough about me to have sex, then I start looking for someone else.

☐ Agree ☐ Moderately Agree ☐ Moderately Disagree ☐ Disagree

TONY, 16-year-old junior. When it comes to sex, I think most people are a bunch of liars. Most guys I know talk like they have sex all the time. I don't believe them. I haven't and I'm 16. I've gone out with a bunch of girls and, yeah, we've messed around, but they never wanted to do it and neither did I. I honestly think the majority of kids haven't actually had sex. They just say they have.

☐ Agree ☐ Moderately Agree ☐ Moderately Disagree ☐ Disagree

JAN, 17-year-old junior. In the first place, sex is over-rated. Secondly, I am sick of guys always wanting to do it. When I was younger, I would give in, but I don't anymore. Hey, if they just want to use my body, they can go hire some prostitute. Don't get me wrong: I like sex, but only with guys who care about *me*. I mean, really, most guys act like sex-starved animals.

☐ Agree ☐ Moderately Agree ☐ Moderately Disagree ☐ Disagree

LISA, 18-year-old senior. You know what I wish? I wish I could find some guy somewhere who really likes me. Not my body. Not my breasts. Just *me*. I wish I could find a guy who cared so much about me that he sent me flowers once in a while and planned some really fun dates. Just once, I wish I could meet a guy who really knew how to talk, not grunt, and who tried to find out all about me. You know? Like, he is actually interested in something besides sports, his car, and his penis?

☐ Agree ☐ Moderately Agree ☐ Moderately Disagree ☐ Disagree

TED, 15-year-old sophomore. OK, I'll admit it. I don't know as much about sex as I pretend. I'm a virgin, yeah, but this sex stuff just gets me all mixed up. I mean, I go out with these girls and they really turn me on, you know. Jeez, they wear halter tops, bikini underwear (you bet I can see it)—they look great. Then when I come on to them, they act like I'm some kind of sex fiend. I mean, what do they expect me to do, sit around and talk about the evening news?

☐ Agree ☐ Moderately Agree ☐ Moderately Disagree ☐ Disagree

KIRK, 17-year-old junior. Hey, I like to go out with girls, OK? I mean, I am normal. But it's like impossible to find a girl who isn't a women's lib type or super-emotional. I'm going with this girl right now. She's great, but I don't want to get serious, OK? I mean, she's always talking about marriage, always freaking out when I talk about going to a college a long way from home. Every time I try to break up with her, she comes unglued, so I back off. I can hardly wait to get out of high school. Hopefully, college girls will be a lot better.

☐ Agree ☐ Moderately Agree ☐ Moderately Disagree ☐ Disagree

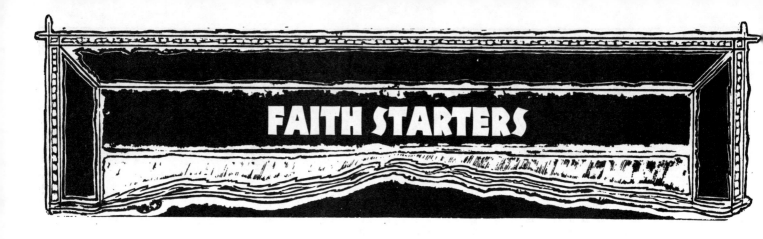

Work with your group to look up as many Bible verses as you can in your assigned category. Read them aloud in your group, and then summarize in your own words what the verses tell us about our sexual behavior.

A Biblical Foundation For Making Decisions In My Life
Proverbs 14:27
Proverbs 28:10
Matthew 6:33
Mark 12:30-31
Romans 12:1-2
Romans 14:19–15:4
1 Corinthians 9:24-27
1 Corinthians 10:31–11:1
Ephesians 4:22-24
Philippians 4:8
1 John 2:15-17

A Biblical Foundation For Making Sexual Decisions In My Life
Job 31:1
Proverbs 7:1-27
Mark 7:18-23
Romans 7:4-6
1 Corinthians 3:16-17
1 Corinthians 5:9-11
1 Corinthians 6:12-20
1 Corinthians 7:8-9, 25-28, 36-38
Galatians 5:16-26
Ephesians 5:1-7
Colossians 3:5-11
1 Thessalonians 4:3-8
Titus 2:11-14

Temptation
Incidents (Genesis 39:1-22; 2 Samuel 11:2–12:23)
Job 31:1
Proverbs 1:10
Proverbs 6:27

Proverbs 7:1-27
Matthew 4:1-11
Romans 6:12-14
1 Corinthians 10:13
Galatians 5:17
Ephesians 6:11-17
2 Timothy 2:22
Hebrews 4:15
James 1:2-16
James 4:7
1 Peter 5:8
2 Peter 2:9
1 John 4:4

God's Opinion of Sex
Genesis 2–4
Song of Solomon

Dating Non-Christians
2 Corinthians 6:14-15

Love
Hosea
1 Corinthians 13:1-13

Marriage
Genesis 2:18-25
Genesis 4:1
Exodus 20:14
Proverbs 5:15-23
Proverbs 6:20-29
Song of Solomon
Matthew 19:1-12
Romans 7:1-25
1 Corinthians 7:1-40

Ephesians 5:22-33
Colossians 3:18–4:1
1 Peter 3:1-8
Hebrews 13:4

Abortion
Exodus 22:22
Exodus 23:7
Psalm 10:8, 14
Psalm 22:3
Psalm 94:6, 20-23
Psalm 139:13-16
Proverbs 6:16-17
Proverbs 24:11-12
Isaiah 49:1
Jeremiah 1:5
Jeremiah 7:6
Jeremiah 22:3

Homosexuality
Leviticus 18:22
Romans 1:1-32
Genesis 19:1-38

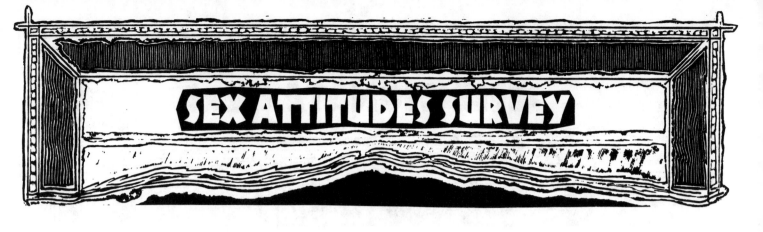

SEX ATTITUDES SURVEY

Please mark each statement "true" or "false."

True   False   1. I know what is right and wrong about sex.

True   False   2. I have a better view of sex than my parents.

True   False   3. If a girl becomes pregnant, it's her fault.

True   False   4. Date rape is wrong under any circumstances.

True   False   5. A person can do anything sexually as long as no one is hurt.

True   False   6. Having sex is a good way to get to know each other.

True   False   7. It is important to marry a virgin.

True   False   8. Very few people wait until marriage to have sex.

True   False   9. Parents should allow kids to make their own sexual decisions.

True   False   10. Sex is overrated.

True   False   11. I know at least one adult I could talk with about a sexual problem.

True   False   12. I don't believe most kids are as sexually active as they say they are. They exaggerate or lie most of the time.

True   False   13. MTV has no effect on my sexual values.

True   False   14. Hard-core pornography is wrong, but *Playboy*, *Penthouse*, and *Playgirl* are okay.

True   False   15. My religious beliefs don't really affect my sexual behavior.

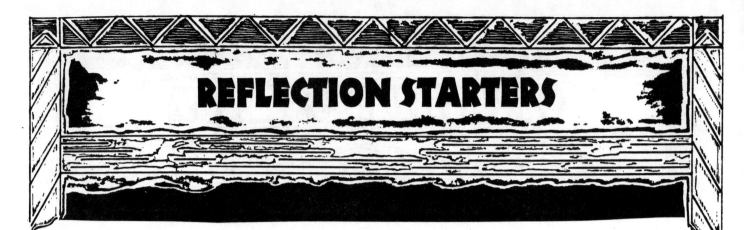

REFLECTION STARTERS

Before the session started, I felt:

During the session I realized:

The most important thing I learned today was:

At the next session I would like to:

I liked the way our leader:

I wish our leader would:

SESSION TWO
VALUES ARE WHERE YOU FIND THEM

Session Purposes

To identify what the media and other influences tell us about sex. To identify popular sexual values and contrast them with Christian values.

Background Brief

Young people can hear sermons, watch videos, and read books on how to have biblical sexual values, but if everywhere except in church they are bombarded with a completely different value system, they don't have a chance. Christian young people need to become aware of the influences in our culture that may be affecting their sexual decisions.

Group Starters

Divide the class into small groups. Give each group a copy of the "Sexual Messages" sheet on page 37 and several magazines, such as *Cosmopolitan, Esquire, Rolling Stone, Spin, People, Time, Sports Illustrated, Vogue,* and *New Woman* (but not obviously sex-oriented magazines such as *Playboy*).

Ask the groups to look at the ads and write down their sexual messages. (Examples: If you use this toothpaste, you will have women crawling all over you. Wearing tight jeans is sexy. Wearing a man's shirt and nothing else turns men on.)

Discuss whether each message is a positive influence or a negative one and whether it's true or false. Ask the young people how they reached that conclusion. Discuss what messages they believe should be communicated by ads regarding sexual behavior and why.

Optional: Have the groups rewrite ads to reflect Christian sexual values.

Alternative activity: Give everyone a copy of the "Society Says . . . " sheet on page 38. Ask them to read each message and mark whether they agree or disagree that today's society is giving us that message through the media, movies, music, or any other source that influences what we think. Discuss as many of the messages as time allows.

Thinking Starters

With the young people in groups, give each person a copy of the "Sexual Influences" sheet on page 39. Ask them to rank each influence to show its importance in shaping their own sexual values and behavior.

Have group members share their rankings with each other and discuss them. What were the reasons for their rankings? Are they happy with the order of influence? See if the group members can agree on the "perfect" order of influence. Who *should* influence you most, etc.? (Don't insist on agreement.)

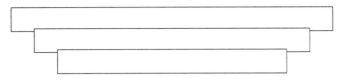

Spend a few minutes discussing the messages sent by the different influences. Do movies, for example, always have a negative influence? Do young people imitate what they see in movies?

Discussion Starters

Here are some ways to use the "Opinions" handouts on page 40:

• Discuss each opinion with the class and try to come to a consensus as to how everyone feels about it. To stimulate discussion, encourage the young people to try to convince the rest of the group that their point of view is correct.

• Have small groups all discuss the same opinion and try to come to a consensus on the agree-disagree scale. Then have each group share its response with the rest of the class.

• Or break into small groups and have each group take a different opinion card and try to reach consensus. Then come back together and ask each group to read its situation and the response. The other groups can react.

• Duplicate the opinion cards and have the young people take them to school and ask others to write their response. At the next session, discuss the responses.

Faith Starters

Divide into six groups and give a different sheet, found on pages 41 through 46, to each group. Or select one verse from the sheets to discuss with the whole class and write it on the board.

Ask each group to rewrite its verse in their own language, making their paraphrasing as modern as possible. (The numbered section on the sheet is for the follow-up activity below.) When the groups are finished, discuss what each verse means today.

Action Starters

Ask volunteers to share what they discovered in this exercise. What could they do to diminish the effect of the negative influences and increase the effect of the positive influences? What decisions could they make regarding their own sexual beliefs and behavior? (Examples: I have decided to cancel my subscription to *Cosmo*. I am not going to take a date to an R movie. I'm going to tell my friends they were wrong about what the Bible says about . . . .)

Alternative activity: (follow up to "Faith Starters") With the young people in six groups, hand out the sheets on pages 41 through 46 with the verses rewritten in modern language. If you use the same groups, give each group a different sheet than they completed earlier. Ask each group to brainstorm three specific sexual behaviors that would illustrate what this verse means.

Have the groups take turns sharing their verses and responses with the class. Then discuss what might happen if they practiced those principles in their daily lives.

Reflection Starters

Ask the young people to share one or two things they learned from this lesson. Then write the question below on the board and ask each person to write an answer.

What areas in my sex life need prayer?

(Example: I just can't see giving up a lot of my sexual behavior. I guess I need help from God to change that attitude.)

Ask them not to sign their names to

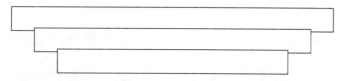

their papers. When everyone is finished, collect the sheets. Remind them that only you will read their papers. Their answers will help you plan the next sessions.

Session Two: Values Are Where You Find Them

In our sexually oriented society we are faced with constant references to sex in television shows, commercials, music, books, ads, and other sources. Our children have grown up surrounded by this, but many are not aware of the values being communicated. They can't recall Lucy and Ricky sleeping in separate beds or Elvis being shown from the waist up.

This session was designed to increase young people's awareness of the values being "taught" by the media and other sources. To help carry over the session at home, after a particularly sensual TV commercial, ask what your son or daughter thought was being "sold." What is the hidden message?

Some evening soon, keep a sheet of paper by the TV and record the number of sexual messages offered in an evening of television, both in the shows and the commercials. Then set aside some time to discuss the following questions with your son or daughter.

Discussion Questions

For parents:
1. When you were growing up, what messages did you get from radio, TV, movies, or advertising regarding
   a. Virginity?
   b. Necking/petting/making out?
   c. Sexual intercourse?

2. What messages did you get from the church or religion regarding these same topics?

For the son or daughter:
1. What messages are you getting from this culture regarding
   a. Virginity?
   b. Necking/petting/making out?
   c. Sexual intercourse?

2. What messages are you getting from our church regarding these same topics?

3. What messages are you getting from us?

4. What can we do to help you with the sexual pressures you are facing?

5. Would you like to talk more about our sexual values?

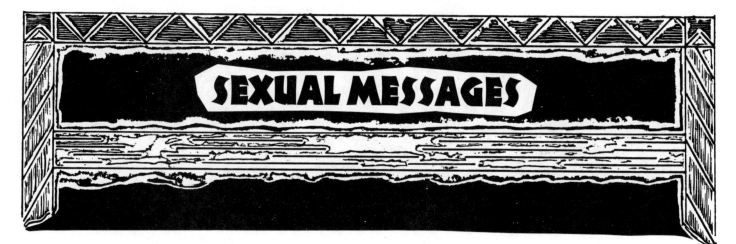

Write down the name of the product and the sexual message the advertisement is communicating. Then evaluate the message. Is it positive or negative? True or false?

Product	Message	Pos/Neg?	True/False?

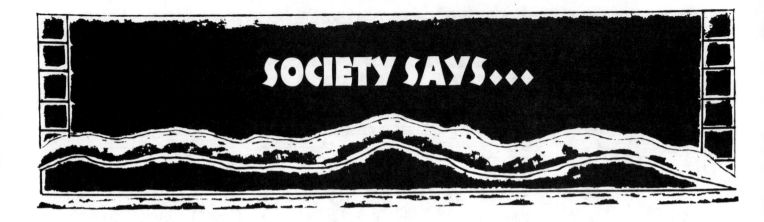

SOCIETY SAYS...

Agree   Disagree   1. Sex is strictly a physical act with no emotional or spiritual consequences.

Agree   Disagree   2. You should have sexual intercourse only with someone you love.

Agree   Disagree   3. Any kind of sexual behavior is okay as long as you practice safe sex.

Agree   Disagree   4. Sexual intercourse is normal and natural between two people who care for each other.

Agree   Disagree   5. Looking sexy is a desirable quality.

Agree   Disagree   6. Being a good sexual performer is one of the most important characteristics you can have.

Agree   Disagree   7. There are no absolute sexual values. You determine what is right for you.

Agree   Disagree   8. Virginity is an undesirable trait.

Agree   Disagree   9. Drinking makes you sexy and desirable.

Agree   Disagree   10. A sporty car makes you sexy and desirable.

Agree   Disagree   11. The kind of perfume/shave lotion you use is sexually stimulating to the opposite sex.

Agree   Disagree   12. Living together is a good alternative to marriage.

Agree   Disagree   13. The more sexual experience you have, the better relationships you will have.

Agree   Disagree   14. It's OK to use sex to make up after a fight, to help yourself or your partner feel better when you are depressed, to "pay" for a nice evening, or to retaliate against someone *as long as you know that's what you're doing.*

Agree   Disagree   15. Without sex, you cannot have a healthy relationship with someone of the opposite sex.

SEXUAL INFLUENCES

Listed below are sources that could influence your sexual attitudes and behavior. Read the list and think about it for a minute. Then number the influences from 1 (most important) to 18 (least important) for YOU.

_____ Parents

_____ Friends

_____ Grandparents

_____ Significant adult

_____ Girlfriend/boyfriend

_____ Siblings

_____ Teacher

_____ Sex Ed.Course

_____ Church

_____ Bible

_____ Pastor

_____ Youth worker

_____ Magazines

_____ TV

_____ MTV

_____ Books

_____ Popular music

_____ Past experience

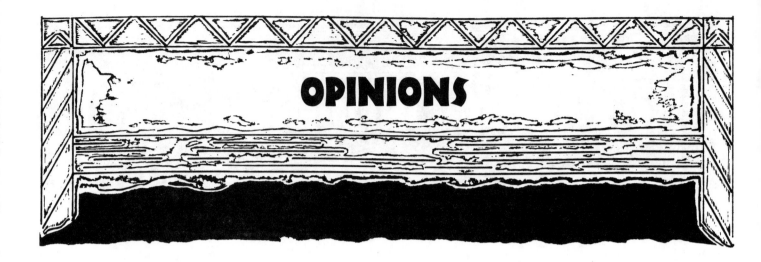

OPINIONS

BILL, 17-year-old senior. I came back from youth group really ticked off. They act like if you watch MTV or look at magazine ads or go to movies, you will end up a sex pervert. Come on! I'm smart enough to know what's wrong and what's right. That stuff doesn't have any influence on me or anyone else. There is nothing wrong with watching anything sexual, except pornography.
☐ **Agree** ☐ **Moderately Agree** ☐ **Moderately Disagree** ☐ **Disagree**

KENNY, 14-year-old freshman. I am so sick of hearing my youth director talk about waiting until marriage and how we're not supposed to kiss, fondle, or do anything except hold hands until we are married. That is so stupid. No one in the entire universe does that except some weirdos. I'll bet you anything my youth director did a lot more than that when she was a teenager.
☐ **Agree** ☐ **Moderately Agree** ☐ **Moderately Disagree** ☐ **Disagree**

CONNOR, 18-year-old senior. They say we're supposed to wait until marriage to have sex. We're supposed to "save ourselves" for marriage. They say that when you wait until marriage, sex is the greatest. Then how come all these adults in my church are getting divorces? How come one of the deacons in our church, the very same deacon who told us to wait until marriage in a Sunday school class, was caught having an affair with a woman in our church? I don't believe waiting until marriage guarantees a happy marriage or great sex.
☐ **Agree** ☐ **Moderately Agree** ☐ **Moderately Disagree** ☐ **Disagree**

KURT, 18-year-old senior. No, I have never had sex or done anything sexual with someone of the opposite sex. I'm glad we talked about all the messages we get from our society because it's true. We do get the message that everyone's doing it and that there's something wrong with you if you don't. Well, I don't and there's nothing wrong with me. Sure it's hard not to, but I pray a lot and I keep myself from getting in too deep. And I'm not ugly, and I'm not weird, and I'm not a prude. A lot of kids would like to think I am so they can justify the fact that they don't want to wait.
☐ **Agree** ☐ **Moderately Agree** ☐ **Moderately Disagree** ☐ **Disagree**

TERI, 15-year-old sophomore. If having a great body doesn't make any difference, then how come everyone I know, including adults in our church, are so freaked out about their bodies? They are all jogging or dieting or working out or taking aerobics or something. I don't care what anyone says, the better your body looks, the better the sex and the better your life.
☐ **Agree** ☐ **Moderately Agree** ☐ **Moderately Disagree** ☐ **Disagree**

CARRIE, 16-year-old junior. You know what I did? I quit watching TV. I quit going to movies. I quit reading dumb magazines and I quit listening to the radio. You know what? It helped. It really did. I can't believe what's happened to me. I read a lot. I think a lot. I have really gotten to know my parents and friends better, and I honestly don't have as much trouble with sex as I used to. It's great. I should have done this a long time ago.
☐ **Agree** ☐ **Moderately Agree** ☐ **Moderately Disagree** ☐ **Disagree**

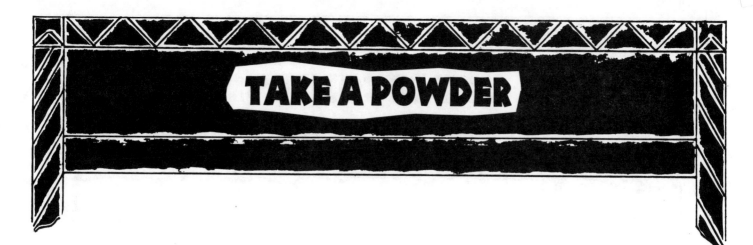

TAKE A POWDER

"Flee from sexual immorality. All other sins a man commits are outside his body, but he who sins sexually sins against his own body. Do you not know that your body is a temple of the Holy Spirit, who is in you, whom you have received from God? You are not your own; you were bought at a price. Therefore honor God with your body" (1 Corinthians 6:18-20).

Rewrite:

Situations where this applies:

1.

2.

3.

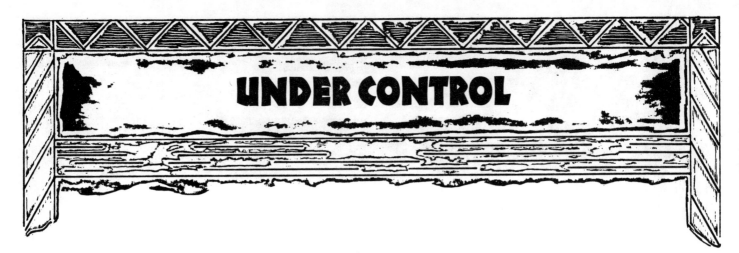

UNDER CONTROL

"It is God's will that you should be sanctified: that you should avoid sexual immorality; that each of you should learn to control his own body in a way that is holy and honorable, not in passionate lust like the heathen . . . " (1 Thessalonians 4:3-5).

Rewrite:

Situations where this applies:

1.

2.

3.

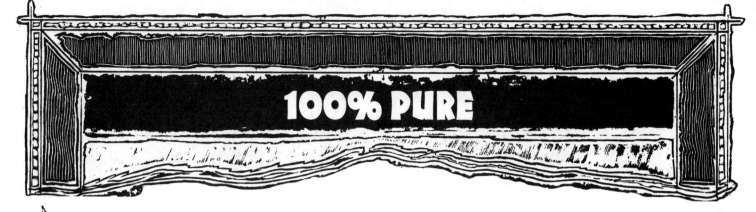

100% PURE

"Marriage should be honored by all, and the marriage bed kept pure, for God will judge the adulterer and all the sexually immoral" (Hebrews 13:4).

Rewrite:

Situations where this applies:

1.

2.

3.

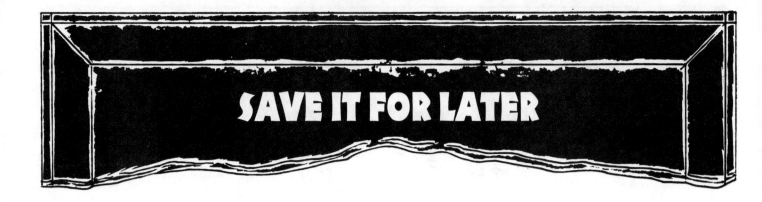

SAVE IT FOR LATER

"Let us behave decently, as in the daytime, not in orgies and drunkenness, not in sexual immorality and debauchery, not in dissension and jealousy. Rather, clothe yourselves with the Lord Jesus Christ, and do not think about how to gratify the desires of the sinful nature" (Romans 13:13-14).

Rewrite:

Situations where this applies:

1.

2.

3.

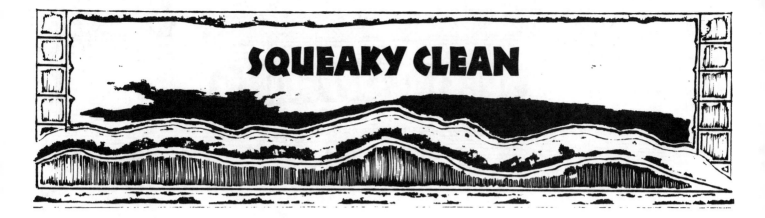

SQUEAKY CLEAN

"But among you there must not be even a hint of sexual immorality, or of any kind of impurity, or of greed, because these are improper for God's holy people. Nor should there be obscenity, foolish talk or coarse joking, which are out of place . . . " (Ephesians 5:3-4).

Rewrite:

Situations where this applies:

1.

2.

3.

SPECIAL OFFERING

"Do not offer the parts of your body to sin, as instruments of wickedness, but rather offer yourselves to God, as those who have been brought from death to life; and offer the parts of your body to him as instruments of righteousness" (Romans 6:13).

Rewrite:

Situations where this applies:

1.

2.

3.

SESSION THREE
MYTHINFORMATION

Session Purposes

To expose myths about sex. To identify and clarify misconceptions some young people have about the Bible's teachings on sexual issues.

Background Brief

Strange as it may seem, this generation of adolescents is not well informed when it comes to sex. Even though most of them have been exposed to sex education courses, they continue to hold firmly to a number of myths about sex. These myths often have a greater effect on their behavior than what they have "learned" in their sex ed courses. This session is designed to expose these myths and to discourage young people from basing their sexual behavior on them.

Your young people may also be confused about some "myths" about biblical sexual values that just aren't true. This lesson provides an opportunity to shed some light on just what the Bible does say about sexual matters. (You may want your pastor or minister to sit in on the "Faith Starters" section to help answer questions.)

Group Starters

Here are three ways to use the "Sex Myths" sheet on page 54:
• Pass out the sheets and have the kids decide which myths are fact or fiction.

When everyone has finished, go back over the list, first comparing answers, then giving the correct answers (which are included at the end of this lesson).
• Ask the kids to look over the "Sex Myths" sheet and as a group decide on the three myths that their friends most commonly believe and that are the most dangerous to a Christian. (If you have a large class, break into smaller groups.)
• After reviewing the sheets, ask the kids to suggest myths that are not listed and discuss those. (Answer only those that you are certain of. Ask a knowledgeable person to answer the others.)

Thinking Starters

Give each student a copy of "Thinking Starters" on page 55 (or write the groups of statements on the board).

Ask the class to read the first group of statements. Choose one or more and ask, "If this was true, how would it change what you do?" Talk about the differences that truth would make in their lives.

Then have the class read the second group of statements. Choose one and ask, "If you really believed that statement, how would it affect your sex life?" (For instance, someone might say, "I wouldn't listen to sex talks because I would figure it will never happen to me." Or for example, someone might say, "I wouldn't worry about how far I went with a guy/

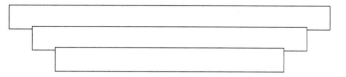

girl because I would always believe I could stop.") Discuss as many of the statements as time allows.

Discussion Starters

Read the "Tension Getter"* below and ask the kids to discuss whether they:

Strongly agree Agree Disagree Strongly disagree

After Sex, Then What?

I had sex with this guy. It wasn't great, but I still liked it. Anyway, I felt guilty about it and I asked God to forgive me. I even broke up with the guy. My youth leaders told me that God did forgive me, and that I should never do it again. I know I shouldn't have sex again, but every time I go out with a new guy, I want to. I can't help it. I've tried to keep from having sex, but once you've experienced it, you can't exactly go back to holding hands. Anyone who thinks you can have sex and then not have it anymore is crazy. Tina, 16-year-old junior

*Reprinted with permission from *Amazing Tension Getters*, Zondervan/Youth Specialties, 1988.

Faith Starters

Pass out the "God Myths" sheet on page 56. Ask the group to decide whether each statement is fact or fiction. Then offer the correct answer. (The answers are included at the end of this lesson, but you may want to have your pastor or minister sit in on this session, too.)

Optional: Have the kids select the three myths most commonly held by their friends and discuss which myth is the most harmful.

Action Starters

Divide the class into small groups and have each one write a talk they would give to teenagers called "What God Wants You to Know About Sex." Have them videotape the talk, if possible, and show it to the group. You might pick the best talk and have it presented to the entire church.

Alternative activity: Have the group write and videotape a commercial that summarizes what they learned in this lesson.

Reflection Starters

Give everyone a copy of "Reflection Starters" on page 57 (or write one or more of the sentence stems on the board). Have the young people complete the sentences. Ask if any volunteers would like to share what they wrote, but be sure not to pressure anyone to share. Collect the papers, if you wish.

Answers for "Sex Myths"

1. Masturbation is perfectly normal and healthy for both male and female.

Fact *and* fiction. Masturbation is normal for both male and female and is practiced by a large percentage of both sexes. But masturbation is not without its negatives. Excess of anything, including masturbation, can cause problems. Excessive masturbation can cause sex to become a very self-centered experience. Sex becomes orgasm-centered and the other person becomes a means to having an orgasm. Excessive masturbation can cause an unhealthy excess of sexual fantasizing. Because something is normal does not mean it is healthy.

2. A girl can't become pregnant:
a. If she has sex during her period. Generally, the ovary releases an egg about two weeks before the menstrual period begins. During the several days it takes to

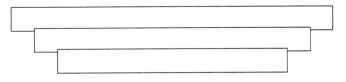

travel down the Fallopian tube, the woman is fertile. The sperm can also live in the Fallopian tubes for several days before the egg is released. Thus, some women can get pregnant for several weeks during their cycle, especially adolescent girls, who often have irregular and unpredictable menstrual cycles.

b. The first time she has sex. If an egg is released, the girl can get pregnant.

c. If she has sex standing up. Gravity has little effect on the sperm even if the girl tries jumping up and down. A girl can get pregnant if she has sex in any position.

d. If she urinates after sex. Remember our biology. Urine doesn't pass through the vagina; it moves through the urethra. Douching or washing out the vagina doesn't work either. You can't wash quickly enough to remove the sperm.

e. Unless the male ejaculates inside her. If a male deposits sperm anywhere near the vagina, the sperm can quickly swim into the vagina with the possibility of fertilizing the egg.

f. If birth control is used most of the time. Birth control must be used *every time* by either the male or female to be effective.

3. If you haven't had premarital sex, you might be gay.

This statement is not only fiction, it is absurd.

4. Lots of sexual experience leads to better marriages.

Sexual experience and/or skill has never been shown to have any positive effect on marriage. In fact, some evidence shows that sexual experience creates problems for marriages because of comparisons and sexual fantasies about the past.

5. Teenagers don't have to worry about sexually transmitted diseases as much as adults.

These diseases can happen to anyone who has sex with an infected person. The incidence of STD among adolescents is *increasing.* In fact, teenagers are more vulnerable to genital infection than adults. The female adolescent's body hasn't matured sufficiently to provide the natural defenses necessary to combat bacteria that may be introduced by the male (Cates, 1985).

6. If you don't have premarital sex, you are impotent or frigid.

Impotency is a man's inability to have an erection. Frigidity is a woman's inability to experience sexual pleasure. Neither impotence nor frigidity has anything to do with premarital sex.

7. If a couple has sex, they will love each other more.

If a couple has sex, they may *feel* like they love each other more, but those feelings are almost always an illusion. Sometimes sex can even become an obstacle to love, because it is used like a drug to blank out real problems in the relationship.

8. Guys need sex more than girls.

Guys may *want* sex more than girls, although that is even questionable, but guys do not *need* sex.

9. Guys don't feel they should be the ones to say "no." They believe the girl should set the standard.

No matter what guys *say*, guys almost always put girls in a situation where they have to say "no." Guys rely on and expect the girl to make the decision.

10. A girl who teases a guy should have sex with him.

Ridiculous. But many girls as well as guys believe that. Girls should not be sexual teases, but whatever they do does not

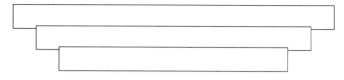

take away their right to say "no" to sex. Nor does *any* girl's behavior give a guy a right to violate her or force sex upon her.

11. If you spend a lot of money on a girl, you should expect some kind of sexual "repayment."

Nonsense. Sex is not something you pay for unless you are with a prostitute. Nothing is more dehumanizing and demeaning than to expect sex for money.

12. If a girl likes you, even though she says "no," she really does want to have sex.

Total nonsense, but a dangerous myth still common among guys. It only perpetuates the macho male ego and is often the justification for date rape.

13. When it comes to sex, guys are basically animals. All they care about is their sexual satisfaction.

This one is fiction, of course, but it is understandable why many would believe it is a fact. Often, guys are afraid to show affection, tenderness, sensitivity, or kindness because they might be called a homosexual. The truth is many guys would like to break out of the male macho image.

14. If you can talk a girl into having sex with you, even though she first said "no," as long as you don't force it, it's not rape.

Force is not just physical, it's also mental. If you manipulate, deceive, verbally abuse, or take advantage of someone so that they allow you to do something they don't want to do, it is wrong.

15. If you love a person, nothing else matters.

If you love a person, everything matters. Love is not an excuse for ignoring your moral standards or personal responsibility.

16. If a girl lets a guy almost completely undress her and then says "no," it's her fault if a guy can't stop.

Absurd. Once again the myth that guys "can't stop" rears it's ugly head. Guys can stop anytime they want to stop. Nothing a girl does takes away from a guy's responsibility for his own actions. Nothing.

17. Just because you spend a lot of time in foreplay doesn't mean that you will have sexual intercourse. Lots of couples spend hours in foreplay and never have sex.

This one is technically a fact. Couples can spend a lot of time in foreplay without having sex, but many couples, if not most, end up having sex. Foreplay leads in only one direction . . . and it isn't Bible reading.

18. You can't go with someone for a long time without increasing your sexual involvement.

This one is technically fiction. You *should* be able to go with a person without getting sexually involved, but it takes a very strong will to do it. Just remember this, if you don't get involved sexually, the sexual pressures are strong, but if you *do* get involved, the sexual pressures will be even worse.

19. If you don't "fool around" on a date, you won't get many dates.

It may be true, it may not be true. If you have a reputation for not fooling around, it may cost you a date with certain kinds of people. On the other hand, some people are relieved to be with a person and not have any sexual pressure.

20. Girls use sex to get love while guys use love to get sex.

This cynical view of sex and relationships is both fact and fiction. Some people are guilty of using sex to get love

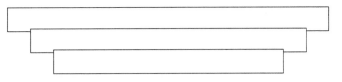

or using love to get sex, but not all people. These kinds of generalizations are destructive because they keep us from recognizing people who do not fit into either category.

Answers to the "God Myths"

1. If you are a good Christian and you accidently go too far sexually, if you pray for forgiveness and really mean it, God will understand and keep you or your girlfriend from getting pregnant.

Nonsense. Being a Christian doesn't guarantee you will not have to experience the consequences of your sin. God certainly can forgive you, and God will certainly be with you, but God will not rescue you from the results of your own choice.

2. If you ask God to take away your sex drive, he will.

For the majority of people, "fiction" would be correct. Sexual drives are God-given, but we cannot count on God to control them. *We* control our sexual drives. God gave us the ability to say "no" and he expects us to use it.

3. Christian adolescents have as much trouble with sex as other adolescents.

Absolutely. Every study that has compared Christian youth to youth who have no practicing faith finds no significant difference in the sexual behavior of the two groups.

4. Once you have sex with someone, the Bible says that makes you married.

The Bible says that the act of sex causes a mystical union between two people, but it does not say that sexual intercourse makes you married (1 Corinthians 6:12-20).

5. Christians believe your sex life is not very important.

Christians are not stupid. They recognize that sex is a powerful force which can unify or destroy people and relationships. Christians believe that the sexual part of our lives is so important that it must be brought under the control of the God who created it.

6. The Bible says it would be better if you didn't get married.

The Bible says that marriage limits your ability to minister. Paul points out that marriage brings with it responsibility and does cause you to reorganize your priorities (1 Corinthians 7). It does not say it would be better if you were not married, period. There is good indication that Paul himself had been married.

7. The Bible doesn't say anything about dating, French kissing, oral sex, masturbation, or sexual foreplay.

True. However, because the Bible doesn't say anything specifically about those things does not mean that it doesn't have plenty to say about how we decide as Christians what to do about specifics. Look up the following Scriptures (also listed under "Faith Starters" in Session 1): Proverbs 7:1-27; 14:27; 28:10; Job 31:1; Matthew 6:33; Mark 7:18-23; 12:30-31; Romans 7:4-6; 12:1-2; 14:19–15:4; 1 Corinthians 3:16-17; 5:9-11; 6:12-20; 7:8-9, 25-28, 36-38; 9:24-27; 10:31–11:1; Galatians 5:16-26; Ephesians 4:22-24; 5:1-7; Colossians 3:5-11; Philippians 4:8; 1 Thessalonians 4:3-8; Titus 2:11-14; 1 John 2:15-17.

8. Christians have the best sex.

Nowhere does the Bible suggest that Christians have the best anything. The Bible does say that if you know Christ, you have life and you know the truth, but it says nothing about the quality of your sex life.

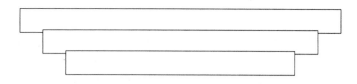

9. Premarital sex is an unforgivable sin.

1 Corinthians 6 points out that sexual sins are unique, but it does not say they are the worst sins—or unforgivable. Sexual sin is like any other sin—it can be forgiven, but the scars will always remain.

10. Sexual desire and lust are the same thing.

Fiction. Sexual desire is normal, natural, and given to us by God. Lust distorts normal sexual desire into abnormal sexual obsession that blinds a person from all moral distinction.

♂ PARENT DISCUSSION GUIDE ♀

Session Three: Mythinformation

Many myths and old tales constantly circulate concerning sexuality. Here are two of them: a girl can't become pregnant if she has sexual intercourse while standing up; if you haven't had sex yet, you might be gay. Most of the mythinformation results from young people getting their "education" from questionable sources, namely their peers. Other problems are caused by the adults in their lives avoiding potentially embarrassing discussions of sex.

Your son or daughter has probably heard these myths and may believe them. To find out—and possibly save considerable grief caused by mythinformation—take a few minutes to discuss the questions below with your child.

Discussion Questions

For parents:
1. How did you learn about sex? From your parents? School? Friends? Church?

2. What were some of the myths about sex going around when you were my age?

For the son or daughter:
1. What is one myth that could cause someone who believes it problems?

2. Do you think the church's view of sex is old-fashioned? Healthy? Helpful?

3. Do you think your mom and/or dad have a good understanding of sex? Be honest!

SEX MYTHS

1. Masturbation is perfectly normal and healthy for both male and female.
2. A girl can't become pregnant:
   a. if she has sex during her period.
   b. the first time she has sex.
   c. if she has sex standing up.
   d. if she urinates after sex.
   e. unless the male ejaculates inside her.
   f. if birth control is used most of the time.
3. If you haven't had premarital sex, you might be gay.
4. Lots of sexual experience leads to better marriages.
5. Teenagers don't have to worry about sexually transmitted diseases as much as adults.
6. If you don't have premarital sex, you are impotent or frigid.
7. If a couple has sex, they will love each other more.
8. Guys need sex more than girls.
9. Guys don't feel they should be the ones to say "no." They believe the girl should set the standard.
10. A girl who teases a guy should have sex with him.
11. If you spend a lot of money on a girl, you should expect some kind of sexual "repayment."
12. If a girl likes you, even though she says "no," she really does want to have sex.
13. When it comes to sex, guys are basically animals. All they care about is their sexual satisfaction.
14. If you can talk a girl into having sex with you, even though she first said "no," as long as you don't force it, it's not rape.
15. If you love a person, nothing else matters.
16. If a girl lets a guy almost completely undress her and then says "no," it's her fault if a guy can't stop.
17. Just because you spend a lot of time in foreplay doesn't mean that you will have sexual intercourse. Lots of couples spend hours in foreplay and never have sex.
18. You can't go with someone for a long time without increasing your sexual involvement.
19. If you don't "fool around" on a date, you won't get many dates.
20. Girls use sex to get love while guys use love to get sex.

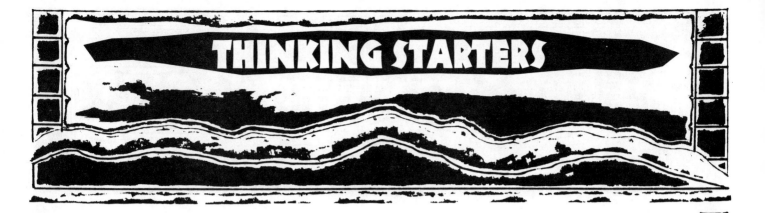

THINKING STARTERS

Group 1:
  a. The world is flat.
  b. The world is going to end in two days.
  c. Certain people have x-ray vision.
  d. There is an elixir you can buy that will keep you young forever.

Group 2:
  a. The more attractive a person is, the better he or she will be in bed.
  b. Once a person has had premarital sex, he or she might as well keep on doing it.
  c. Sex is sacred.
  d. Girls have to say "no" because guys can't.
  e. Pregnancy or sexually transmitted disease will never happen to me or the person I'm going with.
  f. God will stop us before we go too far.
  g. Flirting and talking about sex with someone of the opposite sex is harmless and fun as long as they know you're kidding.

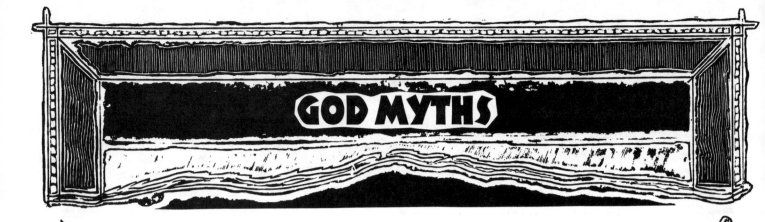

GOD MYTHS

1. If you are a good Christian and you accidently go too far, if you pray and really mean it, God will understand and keep you or your girlfriend from getting pregnant.

2. If you ask God to take away your sex drive, he will.

3. Christian adolescents have as much trouble with sex as other adolescents.

4. Once you have sex with someone, the Bible says that makes you married.

5. Christians believe your sex life is not very important.

6. The Bible says that it would be better if you didn't get married.

7. The Bible doesn't say anything about dating, French kissing, oral sex, masturbation, or sexual foreplay.

8. Christians have the best sex.

9. Premarital sex is an unforgivable sin.

10. Sexual desire and lust are the same thing.

REFLECTION STARTERS

Until this lesson, I never realized that:

I have changed my thinking about:

I believe God wants me to:

I still have questions about:

One thing that surprised me about our discussion was:

SESSION FOUR
PARENTS NEVER HAVE SEX

Session Purposes

To encourage the young people to talk to their parents about sex and understand their parents' sexual values. To give families tools they can use to keep communication open.

Background Brief

It's clear that sex education as now offered in the schools is no substitute for sex education in the home. Nevertheless, most parents have never talked with their adolescents about sex. Really talked. They find it awkward and embarrassing to bring up this sensitive topic. Tragically, especially in the church, parents assume their kids know what their sexual values are, but they don't. One of the most effective solutions to the sexual problems of adolescents today is a dialogue between parent and child. This session was developed to encourage that dialogue.

Group Starters

Divide the class into groups (ideally with an adult in each group) and give each group a copy of "What Should You Do?" on page 62. Have a student in each group read it aloud and lead the group in answering the questions on the sheet.

Thinking Starters

With the young people in the same groups, give each person a copy of "Talk-ing Sex With Your Parents" on page 63.

Have each student go over the list and mark the statement or statements that reflect how they feel about talking to their parents about sex. When everyone is finished, have volunteers share their responses with the group.

Discussion Starters

Have the class brainstorm possible excuses parents might give for not talking to their kids about sex. Now brainstorm ways the *kids* could overcome these obstacles.

Pass out "Who Knows?" on page 64. (Or draw the chart on the board.) Read each numbered statement and have the kids indicate with a show of hands whom they would ask. Total the categories and discuss the pros and cons of the different options.

Faith Starters

Select one or more of the verses below and write it on the board. Discuss with the class what it tells us about talking with parents about sex.

"Children, obey your parents in everything, for this pleases the Lord" (Colossians 3:20).

"Children, obey your parents in the Lord, for this is right. 'Honor your father

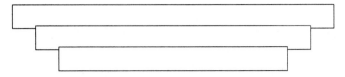

and mother'—which is the first promise—'that it may go well with you and that you may enjoy long life on the earth'" (Ephesians 6:1-3).

"Fathers, do not embitter your children or they will become discouraged" (Colossians 3:21).

"Fathers, do not exasperate your children; instead, bring them up in the training and instruction of the Lord" (Ephesians 6:4).

"A wise son heeds his father's instruction" (Proverbs 13:1).

"Pride only breeds quarrels, but wisdom is found in those who take advice" (Proverbs 13:10).

"Listen to advice and accept instruction, and in the end you will be wise" (Proverbs 19:20).

Action Starters

Give each person a copy of "Helps" on page 65 and discuss the points on it. Then pass out the "Parent Survey" on page 61. Explain that you want each of them to give the survey to their parents. The parents do not have to answer a question if they would rather not, and you can add or subtract any questions you want.

At the next session discuss with the group their overall impressions about talking with parents and list the positive things that came out of this experience.

Reflection Starters

Give everyone a copy of "Reflection Starters" on page 66. Encourage them to complete the sheets and turn them in. Remind them that no one but you will read them.

♂ PARENT DISCUSSION GUIDE ♀

Session Four: Parents Never Have Sex

PARENT SURVEY

Please tell your son or daughter your answers to the questions below. You certainly don't have to answer any question that makes you uncomfortable. Ask your child what he or she thinks about your answers.

1. What are some problems you feel teenagers face today?

2. What are some of your feelings about dating?

3. What is love?

4. When should a couple go steady?

5. Why do teenagers yield to peer pressure?

6. How important is sex in marriage?

7. Is sex overrated?

8. What do you wish your parents would have told you about sex?

9. What are some values you feel would help teenagers make sexual decisions?

10. What do you see as some consequences of premarital sex?

11. What should a person do about his or her sexual feelings?

12. How can a teenager avoid giving in to sexual temptation?

13. What do you think of homosexuality?

14. What are your views on abortion?

15. Do you think teenagers should be allowed to use birth control?

WHAT SHOULD YOU DO?*

Don is 15 and has just started dating Becky. The trouble is, Becky is Don's first real girlfriend and she has, well, been around. Don knows Becky wants to do a lot of things sexually that he isn't sure a Christian should do. He just isn't ready for this, so he decides to talk to someone about the situation. By the way, Becky is the pastor's daughter.

If you were Don, whom would you talk to?
    Your parents?
    Becky's parents?
    Your church youth worker?
    Your best friend?
    Your older sister or brother?
    A good friend who is a girl?

If you wouldn't talk to your parents, why not?

If you would talk to your parents, what makes you think they could handle this discussion?

*Adapted with permission from *Amazing Tension Getters*, Zondervan/Youth Specialties, 1988.

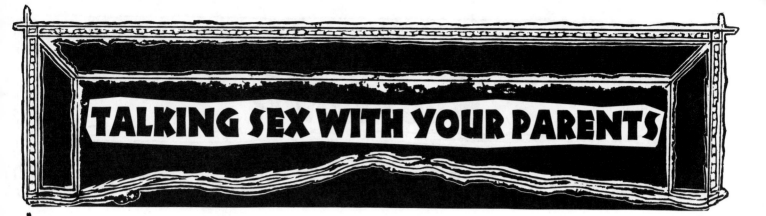

TALKING SEX WITH YOUR PARENTS

Instructions: Can you talk to your parents about sex? Check the statements below that apply.

_____ I can talk to my mother, but no way to my father.

_____ Sex isn't mentioned at my house.

_____ I could talk to my folks, but I won't. Their views about sex are out of the Dark Ages.

_____ I honestly wish they would talk to me, but they don't seem to want to.

_____ My folks are embarrassed about sex.

_____ I think the only time my folks had sex was when I was created.

_____ No way. If I was honest with them about sex, they would lock me up or put me on restriction for the rest of my high school years.

_____ I can't talk with my parents about sex or anything else because they would just get angry if I disagreed with them.

_____ I've tried. All my folks do is joke and tease about sex.

_____ My parents assume it's not necessary to talk about sex because I'd never do anything . . . at least that's what they think.

_____ My parents think *talking* about sex is a sin.

_____ Sure, I talk to my parents about sex. They answer my questions and let me say what I think about it.

_____ I think sex is a private matter and shouldn't be discussed with anyone.

_____ I talked with my parents about sex a while back and now they don't trust me.

_____ I can talk with my parents about anything . . . except sex.

_____ You don't talk with my parents. You just listen.

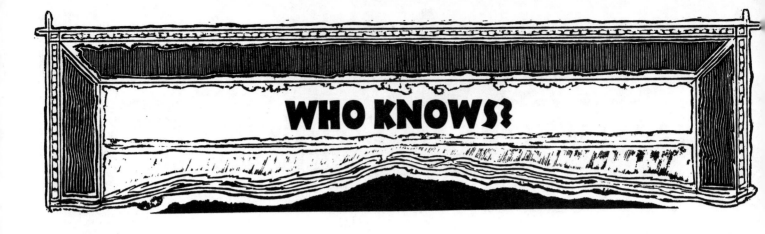

WHO KNOWS?

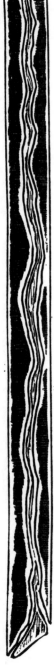

Instructions: Place an X under the person who would be the best to ask about each of the concerns listed.

	girl friend/ boy friend	school counselor	God	Mom	Dad	youth worker/ pastor	friends
How far to go sexually							
What to wear on a date							
Info about birth control							
How to know if you're in love							
Advice about rape/sexual abuse							
Information on abortion							
Where to go on a date							
Questions about masturbation							
Facts about sex							
Confusion over sexual sin							
Who to date							
Concern about pregnancy							

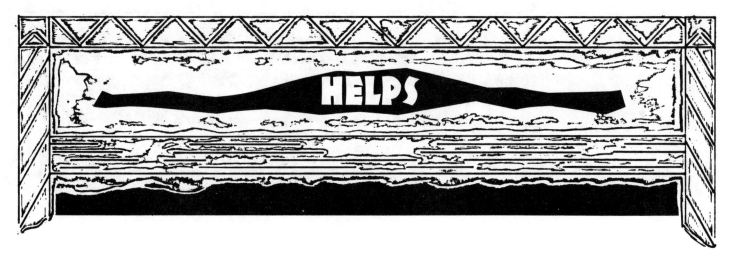

HELPS

Instructions: Try the following suggestions when you talk to your parents.

H ear them out even if you disagree with their views. You want them to hear you, so listen to them. They're concerned about your well-being and really do want the best for you.

E motions are important. Tell your parents how you feel about things. If you're angry about something, let them know. If you are depressed, tell them how you feel. Share your feelings.

L et your parents into your life. It's so easy to exclude them as you become more independent. If you can't think of anything to talk about, share the little things. Don't push them out.

P ray for your parents. They need it just like you do. They also have tremendous pressures upon them. Do it now.

S traight talk is important. Don't beat around the bush. Be as honest as possible.

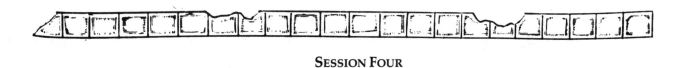

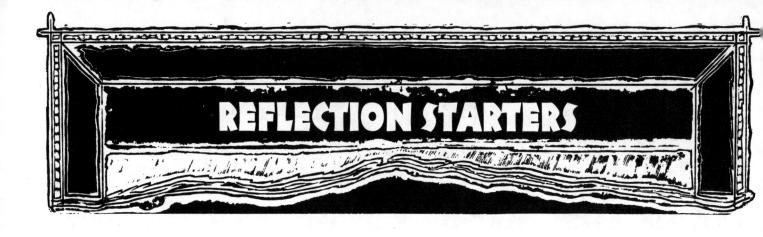

REFLECTION STARTERS

Complete the following questions:

I think that now talking to my parents about sex will be:
    easier   harder   no change

I think the main problem (if there is a problem) my parents and I have when it comes to talking about sex is:

Here's a new thing I have learned about myself:

Here's a new thing I have learned about my parents:

I still would like to know this about my parents:

I wish I could ask God:

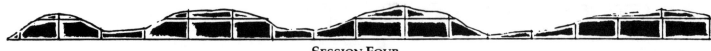

SESSION FIVE
CREATING A REPUTATION

Session Purposes

To explore how we get our reputations and how they can change for better or worse. To discuss the kinds of reputations we would like to have.

Background Brief

Like it or not, young people have sexual reputations, especially in high school and college. In the past having a reputation for being sexually loose was bad. Today, in some circles a bad reputation is good. Young adolescents are confused about what kind of reputation they should create for themselves. Girls and guys want dates with desirable people, but they don't want to be considered a "slut" or an "animal." To evaluate your reputation and consciously try to control or change it as a Christian is a totally new concept and will generate considerable discussion.

Group Starters

Write "reputation" on the board and have the kids brainstorm their definition of it. Compare this to Webster's definition: "overall quality or character as seen or judged by people in general." Guide the class to agree on a working definition of "reputation," combining both versions.

Ask the kids to name slang words that describe someone's reputation. Write them on the board. Are there any positive slang words for someone's reputation? Have the class rank the words they have suggested from best to worst.

Thinking Starters

Before the meeting, select magazine pictures of young people that represent a variety of images (popular, punker, heavy metal, grit, skater, loser, winner, jock, etc.). (Ask the students to help, if you wish.) Tape the photos on the classroom walls and number them.

Have the kids walk around the room and write down a word or words that describe each person's reputation, based solely on the picture. Then take each photo one at a time and ask the class to read their words for it. Discuss why people responded the way they did.

Ask what the people in the pictures have to do with the kids' own reputations.

Discussion Starters

Divide the class into groups and give everyone a copy of "Create-a-Rep" on page 70. Have each group pick a discussion leader and compile a list of positive and negative qualities in each category. For example, for "Body Language," a group might write under Positive "looks at the person who is talking," and under Negative, "flexing muscles, swinging hips."

Have the groups share their responses.

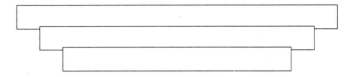

Then ask, "Does a sexual reputation cause the person's behavior *or* does a person's sexual behavior cause his or her reputation?"

Faith Starters

• **Read Galatians 5:19-21 to the group.**
God condemns all of these qualities, but does the society we live in condemn them all as well? Can you think of examples where some of these qualities are encouraged as good?

• **Read Galatians 5:22-23.**
God praises all these qualites as from the Spirit. The verse even says that against all of these there "is no law." If even the laws of a pagan society recognize the goodness of these qualities, why are they so difficult to live out? And why does our society often put down these kind of qualities as wimpish and prudish? (For example: Virginity is looked upon as a negative by many. It's made fun of.)

• **Read Galatians 5:24-25.**
Where does a good reputation come from? Can we all realistically live as Galatians says? If we have a bad reputation, can we change it? How?

Action Starters

Use the "Create-a-Rep" sheets to develop the "perfect" reputation. Select a list of characteristics that would provide a reputation anyone would be proud of.

Afterwards, have each student choose *one* of the characteristics (privately) to practice in his or her own life, beginning now.

If you wish, give everyone a copy of "Rebuilding Your Reputation" on page 71.

Reflection Starters

Give everyone a copy of the "Reflection Starters" sheet on page 72 and ask them to fill it out, without signing their names. Collect them at the end of the session.

♂ PARENT DISCUSSION GUIDE ♀

Session Five: Creating a Reputation

Teenagers are especially concerned about their reputations. No one wants to be thought of as "uncool," "weird," etc. They constantly work on this area of their lives as if they were actors on a stage. As you discuss reputations with your son or daughter, why not pull out the old high school or college yearbook? Tell your child what certain people you knew were like, those with good reputations and with bad ones.

The questions below will help you get started.

Discussion Questions

For parents:

1. What was your reputation when you were in high school? Was it accurate?

2. What was a reputation based on when you were in school?

3. What do you think a reputation should be based on?

4. Do you think reputations are as important today as they were when you were in school?

For the son or daughter:

1. What is your reputation at school?

2. Is it deserved?

3. What would you like your reputation to be?

4. Is there anything we can do to help you have a good reputation?

CREATE-A-REP

With your group, list actions or behaviors for each category that would have a positive influence on someone's sexual reputation. Then list behavior for each category that would have a negative influence.

	Positive	Negative
1. Body Language		
2. Friends		
3. Language		
4. Hangouts		
5. Parties		
6. Music		
7. Clothes		
8. Car		
9. Ways of dancing		
10. Habits		

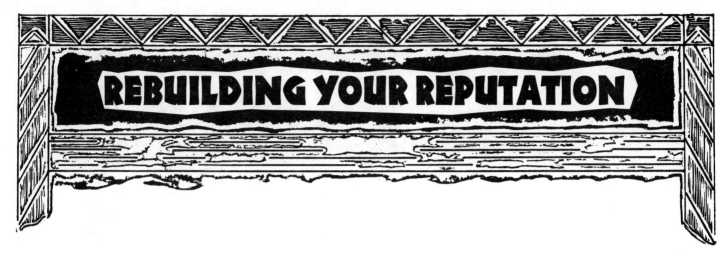

REBUILDING YOUR REPUTATION

DO:

1. Make a clean break with negative friends, hangouts, boyfriends, girlfriends, and activities. Partial breaks are never very successful.

2. Establish a support group, if possible, of adults and kids who can encourage you and be there when the past comes back to haunt you. Obviously, it's easy to say "establish a support group." In reality, it's difficult to make new friends, but church is a great place to start.

3. Live as though your past never happened. Don't deny your past if asked about it, but don't wallow in it either.

4. Let time heal. Some things only time can heal. What you do now will slowly but effectively erase what you did before.

DON'T:

1. Try to convince everyone you've changed. Let your life do the convincing.

2. Let periodic setbacks stop you. Failure is part of recovery.

3. Blame everyone else for your past. Take responsibility for the decisions you made and are making.

4. Get angry at those who continue to hold your past over you. The more you get angry, the more control you give them over you. Ignore them and keep moving on.

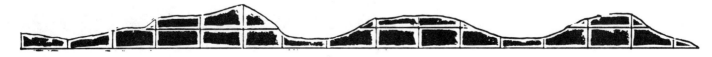

REFLECTION STARTERS

I think my sexual reputation is:
        Great   Okay   No one notices   Uh . . . not great   Awful

I feel my reputation is: Fair   Unfair

The one area I am going to try to change is:

The one question this lesson raised that I still don't understand is:

SESSION SIX
IS DATING DUMB?

Session Purposes

To explore the differences between dating today and in the past. To discuss ways to make dating fun and free of sexual pressure.

Background Brief

Dating was an ancient practice where a guy and girl who did not know each other went together to an activity or event to be part of a group experience, to become better acquainted, or just to have a good time. Dating has changed drastically. Dating is now reserved for couples who know each other, or who have already decided they want to "go together."

It is time for dating to be rediscovered. We believe that healthy dating might be the single most effective solution for helping adolescents resist sexual and relational pressure.

Group Starters

Read aloud "Ancient Dating" on page 76 and ask the kids whether it sounds good, bad, corny, boring, etc. Do they wish ancient dating was practiced today?

Now ask what they like and don't like about modern dating. Do they think modern dating creates more sexual pressure on kids than ancient dating did? Why or why not?

Some people suggest that nearly 50% of the kids in high school never have a date.

Do your young people believe that's true? What's wrong with not dating in high school?

Optional: Ask your group to survey the college age, single adult, or adult Sunday school classes to see how many of them dated in high school. Discuss the results in class.

Thinking Starters

Divide the class into groups and give everyone a copy of "Rent-a-Date" on page 77. Have each person decide how he or she would spend the $25. Then have the kids share their decisions in the small groups.

Afterwards, discuss these questions with the class:

• What kind of person should we date? Does it matter?

• Should we date with the view that anyone we date could end up being our mate?

You can also use and discuss the optional "Dating Pros & Cons" sheet on page 78. Using the sheet, have your kids list the pros and cons of dating. Next, list on a blackboard the specific components of a typical date and have your kids discuss the pros and cons of each component.

Discussion Starters

Pass out the "Creative Dating" sheet on page 79, stolen from *Creative Dating* by

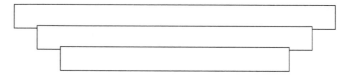

Doug Fields and Todd Temple, Oliver Nelson Publishing. See if the class can come up with ten creative dates.

Afterwards, talk about how much fun it was coming up with the ideas and how the focus of the date shifted to the date itself, not the people on the date. Point out that the more creative the date, the less sexual pressure there is on the people who are dating. When a date is fun, the pressure for intimacy is less.

Faith Starters

Read Romans 12:1-2 and Philippians 4:8-9.

Obviously, neither of those passages says anything about dating. In fact, the entire Bible doesn't say anything about dating. Point out that when talking about sex and dating, people often get too spiritual. That's right, too spiritual. Ask the kids if they can summarize in two simple sentences what those two verses say about the way we live our lives.

Point out that one way we can keep from being "conformed to this world" is by "transforming" the way we date. Instead of a date being a pressure-filled, sexually-explosive experience, as committed Christians, we can make dates fun, creative, positive experiences with minimum opportunities for sexual sin.

Action Starters

Option One: This is a totally wild and risky idea, but try it anyway. Plan a group date. Have the entire group plan an evening, afternoon, morning, or the whole day together. Remember, this is a date, not a field trip, so plan the time so you can get to know each other and experience things together. After the date, discuss what happened. Was anyone surprised at how much fun it was?

Option Two: For their next date, have the kids suggest a box lunch picnic or some other creative alternative. Suggest that guys or girls ask out someone they don't know, but want to. See what happens.

Option Three: Ask the kids to write a "New Year's Resolution" on dating, including what they will and won't do and what types of people they will and won't date.

Reflection Starters

Give everyone a copy of the "Reflection Starters" sheet on page 80 and ask them to think about the session for a minute before answering the questions. Collect the completed sheets, if you wish.

Session Six: Is Dating Dumb?

Open this discussion with your son or daughter by describing what dating was like when you were younger. Did anyone ever really call and ask a relatively unknown acquaintance for a date? Did people really go on blind dates? Why?

For those parents who are now in dating situations: your son or daughter is learning dating behaviors from you. Talk with him or her about your dating. Explain what you think are essentials for a good date. The questions below will also help you and your young person share your thoughts and feelings.

Discussion Questions

For parents:

1. What was dating like when you were in high school?

2. What was the best date you ever had? The worst?

3. Did you like dating?

4. Would you like to see me date more? Or less?

5. Would you help me plan some wild and creative dates?

For the son or daughter:

1. Why do you think kids don't date as much as they used to?

2. Is there anything you don't like about dating?

3. If you have dated, do you like it? If you haven't, does it bother you?

ANCIENT DATING

Many years ago young men and women practiced an ancient ritual called dating. The male talked to a female at school or on the way home from school. When the male was sure the female knew who he was, he would call and ask her to go out on a "date." The date might involve going to a dance or movie. The boy and girl would attend the entire event together, go out afterwards for a Coke and fries, and then go home, usually pretty early. Often the dates were during the day and involved a picnic or an afternoon at a park.

Almost always, the female would have to get permission from her parents first, and the male would have to meet her parents before the date. Dating was practiced by kids who were at least 16, and the male asked the female, never the other way around. Most dates were "double dates," with two couples. Very little sex, if any, was involved. Usually there was lots of talking, holding hands, an arm around the girl, and maybe a kiss at the door.

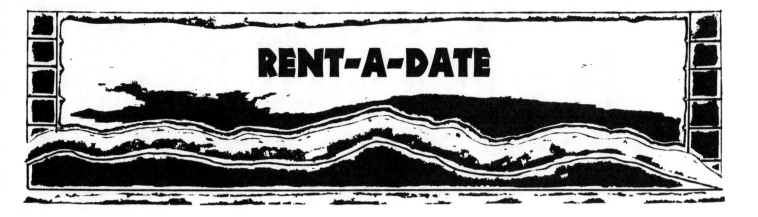

RENT-A-DATE

You get to "Rent-a-Date." You have $25 to spend. Listed below are a number of qualities, each marked with a price. Look over the list and decide how you want to spend your money.

Attractive body ($6)

Romantic ($3)

Wise ($2)

Great hair ($2)

Good manners ($2)

Well groomed ($2)

Athletic ($1)

Tall ($1)

Popular ($6)

Committed Christian ($6)

Virgin ($6)

Kind and considerate ($5)

Great at kissing ($5)

Good-looking face ($5)

Sense of humor ($5)

Intelligent ($5)

Sexy ($4)

Goal-oriented ($4)

Friendly ($4)

Owns a car ($3)

Fun ($3)

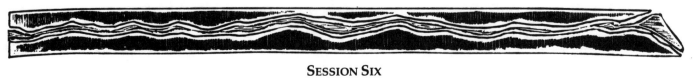

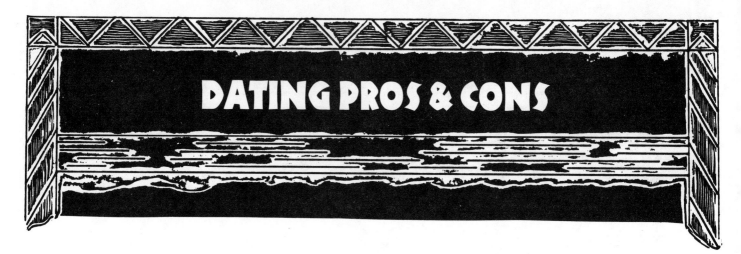

DATING PROS & CONS

	Positive (benefits)	Negative (dangers)
Age:		
Under 14		
15-16		
16-19		
Girl 14, guy 18		
Girl 17, guy 21		
Guy 16, girl 18		
Car dating		
Prom date		
Double dating		
Grad night		
Weekend camping or skiing		
Home, no parents		
Friend's house, no parents		
Jacuzzi date		
All day at beach		
Party		

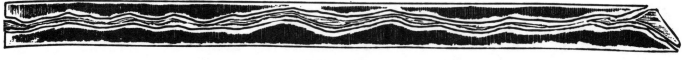

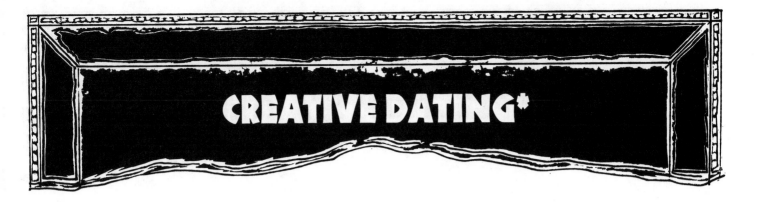

CREATIVE DATING*

1. Go to Slip 'n' Slide together.

2. Have dinner by candlelight at McDonald's.

3. Tour a golf course in a golf cart.

4. Build a sand castle together.

5. Mission Impossible: Mail instructions that will eventually lead your date to you and the rest of the evening's activities.

6. Random Pictures: Take pictures of places to go and things to do. Put each picture in a separate envelope and then have your date pick one. Go to that place, then have your date pick the next photo.

7. Tourist Night (or day): Dress like outrageous tourists and spend the day or evening doing touristy things.

8. Friend-ly Date: Invite a bunch of your friends to help you take your date "out" to dinner—at your house or a park. Have a friend dressed as a valet park your car, another friend bring you to your table (prepared by you ahead of time), another friend wait on you, etc.

9. Ballroom dancing: Sign up for dance lessons with your date to learn the fox trot, samba, rhumba, and tango.

* Adapted with permission from *Creative Dating*, Fields & Temple, Oliver Nelson Publishers, 1988.

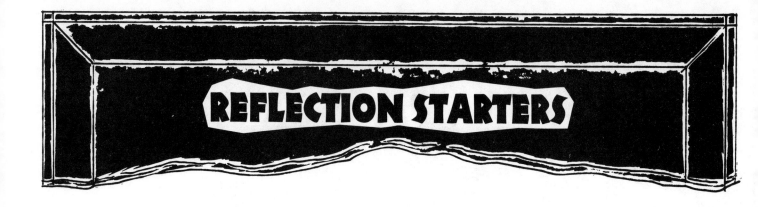

REFLECTION STARTERS

When it comes to dating . . .
_____ I am more frustrated than I was
_____ Less frustrated than before
_____ No change
Why?

If I do the following, my social life will be better:

If I'm honest . . .
_____ Creative dating may help relieve sexual pressure.
_____ Creative dating won't make any difference.
Why?

The one spiritual lesson I've learned from this session is:

I still have a question about:

I wish God would give me the strength to:

SESSION SEVEN
GETTING SERIOUS

Session Purposes

To explain why some kids "get serious" and why it's so dangerous. To help the young people develop a plan for never getting serious.

Background Brief

For the kids who are "going with someone" in high school, the process of choosing a lifetime partner is already in trouble. Many adolescents get seriously involved sexually with someone long before they know who that someone is. They confuse sexual intimacy with real intimacy and often end up marrying a total stranger.

They need to understand that high school is the worst time to decide on anything permanent, especially a marriage partner. Most kids who are seriously involved in high school feel the pressure of their relationship and would like to get out, but don't know how without hurting the other person. It's time to give adolescents the ammunition they need to get out of serious relationships and stay out until they are old enough to make lifetime decisions. The problem of Christians and non-Christians getting serious will also be discussed.

Group Starters

Pass out "Why Get Serious?" on page 84 and discuss each reason given. Are they valid? Are there other reasons besides the ones on the list?

Now give everyone a copy of "A Letter from Darla" on page 85. Do they agree or disagree with what she said?

Thinking Starters

Pass out copies of the "Quiz on Relationships" on page 86 and ask the kids to complete it. Explain that you aren't going to collect it and no one else will see their answers, but the quiz may help them decide whether their relationships are getting too serious. After everyone is finished, ask volunteers to respond to the quiz.

Alternative activity: Set up a debate. Have one side argue that getting serious is the only way to go. Have the other side argue that staying away from serious relationships is much healthier.

Discussion Starters

Say to the group:

Let's pretend you decided never to get serious with anyone in high school. What are the rules you would live by to ensure you didn't get serious?

Have the group brainstorm rules. Then ask if, after developing the list of rules, they think it's possible to go through high school without getting serious. Why or why not?

Sample rules:

1. I would never date a person more than _____ times.

2. I would always have the person meet and talk with my parents.

3. I would ask my friends to nail me if I was getting too serious.

4. I would group-date a lot.

5. On alternate weekends I would do things with my friends and have no dates.

Faith Starters

It's time to ask the killer question. Should Christians date non-Christians? Or just Christians? Just any Christians? Only committed Christians?

Read 2 Corinthians 6:14-16. Ask the kids to give their interpretation of those verses. You might clarify the passage with the following explanation:

The apostle Paul uses the metaphor of the double yoke, which was used to hold two oxen side by side while they worked the fields. Paul is not condemning all contact with non-Christians, but he is saying that close, serious relationships should involve believers only. However, this Scripture does *not* mean we are to separate ourselves from society.

Now ask the group if they think the double yoke applies to marriage, engagement, going steady, casual dating, close friendships, or casual friendships.

Conclude by asking the group to identify the kinds of people God would want them to date.

Action Starters

Have each person devise an action plan on one of two subjects:

• "How To Keep Myself From Getting Serious" (Example: I will never date one person exclusively.)

• "How To Keep Myself From Getting More Serious" (Example: I will make sure that every date is planned with no more than 30 minutes to get home.)

Have volunteers share their action plans with the group.

Reflection Starters

Give everyone a copy of "Reflection Starters" on page 87 (or write some or all of the sentence stems on the board). Ask the students to finish the sentences. If you wish, collect the papers.

♂ PARENT DISCUSSION GUIDE ♀

Session Seven: Getting Serious

In this session we discussed the value of dating several people versus "getting serious" with someone. The questions below will help your child think about the consequences of getting serious too soon, both sexually and socially.

Discussion Questions

For parents:

1. How old were you when you first were "serious" about someone?

2. How did you know when you had found the right person to marry?

3. (If parents are divorced) Knowing what you know now, what would you have done differently in choosing your first husband/wife?

4. Do you think I should just date Christians?

For the son or daughter:

1. What do you think is the minimum age to get serious?

2. What do you look for in a guy/girl?

3. How will you know when you meet "Mr./Ms. Right"?

4. What do you think are some advantages of getting serious with someone? Some disadvantages?

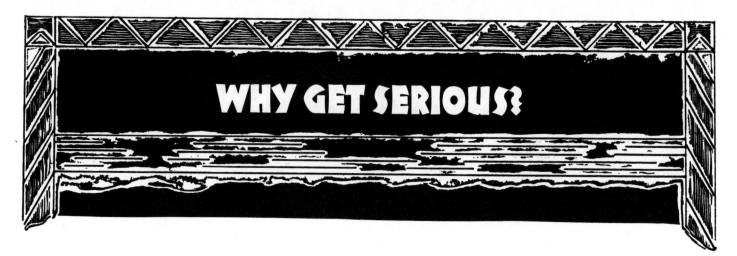

WHY GET SERIOUS?

1. You don't have to worry about who will be your next date.

2. It feels good to know Mr./Ms. Wonderful likes only you.

3. It makes you feel desirable. You always wondered if anyone would ever like you enough to get serious, so when someone does, it feels real good.

4. Pride. You've landed the big fish a lot of other people would like to have.

5. You can quit worrying about how you eat and what to say. You get comfortable with a person and that takes the pressure off. It's like he or she is part of the family.

6. You have someone you can confide in. You have someone to spout off to when you get into it with your parents or another friend, or you're having trouble in school.

7. One of the big problems in high school is loneliness. When you have a steady boyfriend/girlfriend, you are seldom alone.

8. It's fun! It's great to have someone you can do things with who is so familiar. It's a lot more fun to spend time with a friend than a stranger.

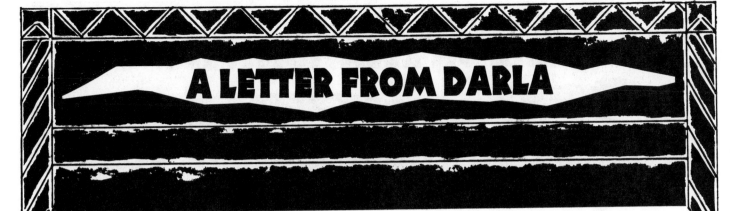

Get serious with a guy? Forget it! The day I decided to quit getting serious was the best day of my life. Going steady with someone is horrible. It's your worst nightmare. They act like they *own* you. You have to explain your every movement. They tell you how to dress, how much make-up to wear, how to fix your hair. They want to know where you are at every second. They get jealous all the time, even of your friends! (How come you were talking with Eddy? Someone told me they saw you walking with Darrell.)

They dictate what you can do when you're with them and when you're not with them. They get mad if you go someplace where there are guys you could meet. And the macho bit! They are always making you choose between something and them. You know, like an ultimatum. It's either your friends or me! It's either Young Life camp or me!

Can you believe I put up with that stuff? The last guy I was serious with told me it was either him or the Mexico trip our church was doing and I said, "That's fine with me. I'm going to Mexico." He couldn't believe it. And most of them don't like your parents. They don't like to talk with them or go anywhere with them. All the guys I went with caused so much grief with my parents, and I let these jerks do it.

And the sexual pressure! I can't believe how many hours I sat around with various boyfriends talking about sex! Should we or shouldn't we? How come I didn't want to? I hurt his feelings! What about my feelings? I got sick of being treated like a thing. He would get mad, threaten me, even. Try to force me to have sex and then, get this, tell me I liked being forced.

Let me tell you, the best thing I ever did was get my freedom back. Now, I date guys when and if I want to. I spend time with my friends, my family. I dress how I want and go where I want. I love my freedom. And don't get me wrong. I like to date guys, but I want to enjoy high school. I want to experience everything I can without having some slave-master telling me what to do.

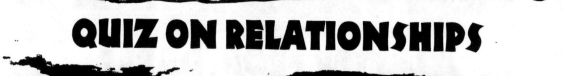

QUIZ ON RELATIONSHIPS

_____ 1. Do we talk about things that matter? (not just sex, football, and next week's party) Yes-10, No-0

_____ 2. Do we have fun together? Yes-10, No-0

_____ 3. Do we argue all the time? Yes-0, No-10

_____ 4. Do we argue about sex all the time? Yes-0, No-10

_____ 5. Is sex the only good thing about our relationship? Yes-0, No-10

_____ 6. Do I feel trapped and secretly wish I weren't so tied down? Yes-0, No-10

_____ 7. Do I secretly wish I could date someone else? Yes-0, No-10

_____ 8. Are there lots of differences between us? Yes-0, No-10

_____ 9. Do either one of us have a problem with jealousy? Yes-0, No-10

_____ 10. Is the spiritual part of our life important to both of us? Yes-10, No-0

_____ Total

SCALE: 70-100   Sounds like a healthy relationship
         50-70   Okay relationship
         20-40   You've got problems
         0-10   You've got serious problems

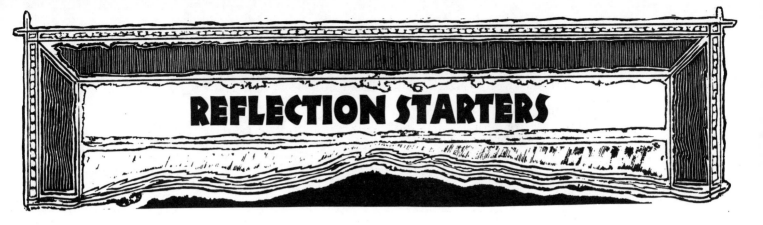

REFLECTION STARTERS

The most difficult thing I learned during this lesson was:

I want to change, but the area I find most difficult to change is:

I heard some things I know are true, but I don't want them to be true. Here is a list of those things:

Please pray for me about:

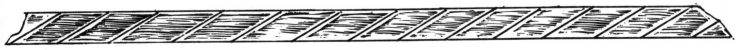

SESSION EIGHT
HOW TO SAY "NO" WHEN YOU WANT TO SAY "YES"

Session Purposes

To introduce a four-step plan to say "no" to sex. To identify the kinds of sexual temptations young people encounter. To name positive activities to replace those temptations.

Background Brief

Adults often have trouble understanding why adolescents can't "just say no" to sexual temptations. A lot of those adults have forgotten what it's like when your hormones are on overload. It is not easy being an adolescent in a "sexualized" world. Thus, refusal is more than saying "no." It is a process that involves specific skills.

The first skill is identification. Adolescents must be able to identify the temptation they are facing. The second skill, personalizing, is the ability to recognize the consequences if you don't say "no." The third skill is option-making. Adolescents must be able to think of options to say "yes" to, so they don't say "no" in a vacuum.

If young people learn the first three skills, the fourth, invitation, is much easier. Adolescents must be able to walk away from a negative situation into a more positive one and bring others with them. Saying "no" does not have to mean the loss of friends; it can mean that friends say "yes" together to other activities.

Group Starters

Pass out copies of "You Would If You Loved Me" on page 93 or write some of the "lines" on the board. Point out that both guys and girls use these lines. For each one, ask the group to brainstorm clever comebacks. What other lines have they heard people use to get sex?

Ask why people use lines on each other. Do lines actually work? Why or why not? Which lines are the most difficult to refuse?

Point out that no one would need lines if the other person wanted to do what he or she was being asked to do. Lines are manipulative and exploitive. But they often work because, the better you know a person, the better you know how to play on their weaknesses.

Thinking Starters

Have a guy and a girl role play a situation in which one of them uses a line and the other one says "no" in a creative way. When the guy/girl says the line, someone standing nearby will say what the person is really thinking. Before the other person says "no," another voice will say what that person is really thinking.

Here's an example:

GUY: Look, we've been going together now for a month. It's obvious we're going to be together for a long time. We

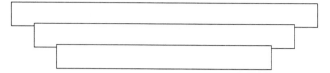

feel so close now so why not have sex? It will bring us even closer together.

VOICE 1: What's the point of going together all this time if we're not having sex? If she doesn't come through, I'm breaking this off.

VOICE 2: He has really been putting pressure on me lately. If I don't come across, I'll probably lose him. I don't want to lose him, but I don't want to have sex either. Hmmmmmmm. I know what I'll say . . .

GIRL: I want to be close, but I've been hurt so many times in the past I just need more time. Let's enjoy each other without adding the pressure of sex right now.

Have the group evaluate how realistic the role play was. In the above example, did the girl leave herself open to even greater pressure later? Was there something else she could have said?

Discussion Starters

(This section introduces the four-step process to saying "no" to sex.)
1. Ask the group to **identify** all the tempting sexual situations they can think of so you (or a volunteer) can write them on a list. Be specific and realistic. The list could include anything from watching a porno flick to receiving or writing a suggestive note in class. Combine similar temptations.
2. Now have the group **personalize** the temptations on the list. That simply means asking, "What would be the consequences if I did that?"
3. Now brainstorm **options** to each situation on the list. What positive things could you do in that situation? Be as creative and realistic as possible.

Explain that the group has just completed three of the four steps necessary to say "no." Give everyone a "Know How" sheet on page 94 and review the steps, especially the fourth one. Mention that at times they may have no choice but to lose a friendship or a relationship.

Faith Starters

Ask a volunteer to read Genesis 39:1-23 aloud. Discuss it with the group, bringing out the following points:
• Potiphar's wife limited her relationship with Joseph to the physical dimension (Genesis 39:7).
• Joseph repeatedly refused her sexual advances even to the point of avoiding her (Genesis 39:10).
• Joseph overcame temptation in spite of his vulnerable situation (Genesis 39:10).
• Joseph was able to refuse Potiphar's wife's advances, but finally he had only one way out. He ran. Resisting or running are two good ways to overcome temptation (Genesis 39:11-12; 2 Timothy 2:22; James 4:7).
• Joseph was willing to face the consequences of his decision. He traded his good situation for a bad one—prison. It would have been much easier for Joseph to give in, yet he refused (Genesis 39:19-20).
• Joseph's decision was based on his relationship with God and the values he held as a result of that relationship (Genesis 39:2, 21, 23).

Ask the group how Joseph's life would have been different if he would have given in to Potiphar's wife. Did saying "no" hurt Joseph? How did saying "no" pay off for Joseph? Why do they think Joseph had the strength to say "no"?

Action Starters

Read each situation below and ask the group what they would do. Then apply

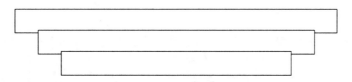

the four "K<u>no</u>w How" steps to the situation.

• A boyfriend/girlfriend, after an evening together, tries to kiss you, but you are not ready. Do you . . .
  1. Go ahead and kiss because it's expected.
  2. Tell the person you aren't ready.
  3. Say something like "Uh . . . I'd like to, but my lips are chapped."
  4. Other

• You are kissing and the guy tries to slip his hand in your blouse, or the girl puts your hand on her breast. Do you . . .
  1. Go for it.
  2. Move his hand away, or move your hand off her breast.
  3. Stop everything and take a breather.
  4. Other

• You are at a party with a person you like but don't want to get serious with. Everyone starts making out. Do you . . .
  1. Join in but not wholeheartedly and hope you can get out of this soon.
  2. Tell your date you have mono.
  3. Leave the party.
  4. Other

• You are going out with someone you really like, except he or she always wants to make out, even in public. Do you . . .
  1. Give an ultimatum. "Cool it or we break up."
  2. Use reverse psychology and grope your partner in front of friends or parents.
  3. Ask the person's best friend to talk to him/her.
  4. Other

• After school, you stop by your girlfriend/boyfriend's house. You didn't realize no one else would be home. The two of you have gone a little too far sexually with each other in the past. Do you . . .
  1. Leave
  2. Stay, but go outside in the front yard where you can be seen.
  3. Stay. Nothing will happen because someone may come home any minute now.
  4. Other

Here are some extra tips to give the group:
• Set your sexual standard right now rather than later in the back seat of a car or in another compromising situation.
• Once you set your standard, stick with it.
• Find friends with similar beliefs and support each other in your values and decisions.
• Understand you don't have to give a reason when you say "no." It's your body. You make the decisions.
• Be aware that the further you go sexually, the easier it is to keep going. Physical intimacy will inevitably lead to more of the same.
• Don't put yourself in compromising situations.
• Find other ways to express your feelings for each other.
• Guys, as well as girls, need to say "no."
• If you're not happy with what you are doing, talk it over with an adult you trust.

Reflection Starters

Give everyone a copy of "Reflection Starters" on page 95 (or write the sentence stems on the board). Ask them to think quietly about the sentences for a minute and respond to each one. Explain that you won't be collecting the papers today, but you want them to think about these topics.

♂ PARENT DISCUSSION GUIDE ♀

Session Eight: How to Say "No" When You Want to Say "Yes"

When your son or daughter was growing up, you might have said, "Kiss Grandma goodbye," and so on, but now our teenagers have to decide who they will kiss and who they will touch. We want them to "just say no," but they have to know *how* and *why* to say it.

Let your son or daughter know you were normal and struggled with this area too when you were younger. (Spare the morbid details, but share the frustration.) Discuss ways they could get out of some difficult situations. Encourage them to blame it on you by saying something like, "My parents won't allow me to get serious with someone."

Your son or daughter is making critical decisions. Deciding how and why to say "no" will be the best preparation for times when the situation arises, and it always does!

Discussion Questions

For parents:

1. Do you have a hard time saying "no" to people?

2. How do you say "no" when you want to say "yes"?

For the son or daughter:

1. When do you find it most difficult to say "no"?

2. What have you learned in this lesson about saying "no"?

3. Do you believe God can help you say "no"?

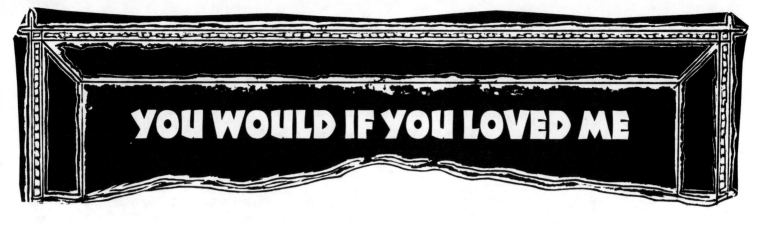

YOU WOULD IF YOU LOVED ME

1. You are so lucky to be out with a person like me.

2. All my friends are doing it.

3. We won't go all the way.

4. I have never met a woman (or man) like you before.

5. You must be a homosexual (frigid) if you don't want to do anything.

6. I will show you how to do it.

7. It will make a woman (man) out of you.

8. I want to marry you some day, so why not?

9. Nobody has ever really cared or loved me like you have.

10. Prove you love me.

11. I will still respect you.

12. Trust me. I know what I'm doing.

13. But I love you!

14. No one will ever know.

15. I love you. Don't you love me?

16. But it feels so right.

17. You don't know what you're missing!

18. You can't get pregnant this time of the month.

19. It will bring us closer together.

20. I have never loved anyone like I love you.

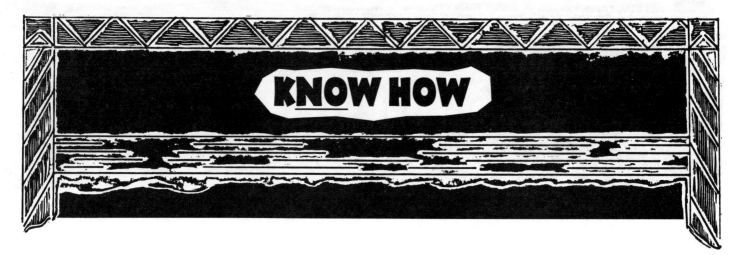

KNOW HOW

1. **Name the Temptation.**

   "He wants me to have sexual intercourse."
   "She wants to get undressed."

2. **Personalize the Temptation.**
   What are the consequences if you give in?

   "If I did that, I might get pregnant."
   "If I did that, I would lose my self-respect."
   "If I did that, I would be tempted to go further."

3. **Find Things to Say "Yes" To.**
   Suggest something positive to do instead.

   "Let's go to the mall."

4. **Extend an Invitation.**
   Ask your friend or friends to join you in the new activity.

   "I'm going to the mall. Why don't you come with me?"

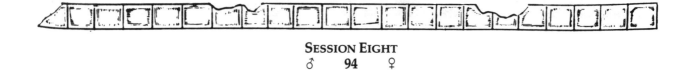

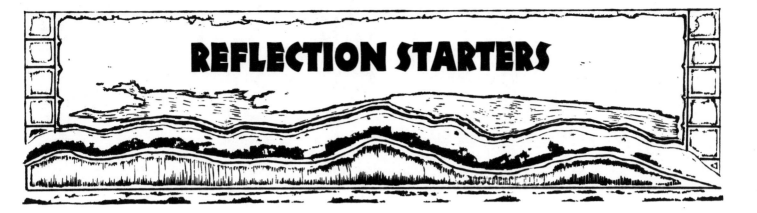

REFLECTION STARTERS

When it comes to saying "no" about sex . . .
    _____ I have no problem
    _____ It depends on whom I'm with
    _____ I have lots of problems

I need to say "no" when:

If God can really help me in this area, I just have one question for him:

Today I learned:

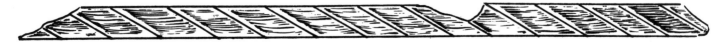

SESSION NINE
HOW FAR SHOULD YOU GO?

Session Purposes

To teach that values don't just happen: they are conscious decisions we make. To help adolescents decide their sexual standards.

Background Brief

Although the Bible is clear about fidelity in marriage and chastity outside of marriage, it is painfully silent on the specifics of sexual conduct before marriage. The Bible doesn't mention kissing, giving hickeys, fondling sexual organs, or engaging in oral sex. Unfortunately, many adolescents find themselves struggling with those very issues. The old adage "save sex until marriage" has been replaced by "be responsible with sex until marriage."

Our culture seems to have abandoned chastity as a viable option for adolescents, but the church has not. Still, when society encourages a low sexual standard, it is difficult for young people to maintain a higher one. They have to decide against the majority of their friends, our culture, and the pressures created by their own sexual development.

That's why it's vital that adolescents receive help and encouragement to practice a high sexual standard. Notice that the title of this session is not "How far *can* I go?" but "How far *should* I go?" The question is not "What can I get away

with?" but rather "How can I take control of this volatile area of my life?" This session does not tell the young people what to do, nor does it suggest that it doesn't matter what they decide. Instead, it encourages them to decide now what they will do later, keeping biblical principles in mind.

Group Starters

The two surveys—"Premarital-Sex Quiz" on page 100 and "Petting Quiz" on page 101—will help your group explore some important decisions about how far they should go in their sexual relationships. Look both quizzes over and decide which is appropriate for your group. (Perhaps the "Petting Quiz" on page 101 might be more suitable for a younger group.)

Give everyone a copy and have the kids mark each statement "Agree" or "Disagree," without signing their names to the papers. Then complete the activity with either of these options:

Option 1: Discuss all the statements or ask the group which ones they'd like to talk about. (If your group is shy, ask everyone to write the numbers of two or three statements they'd like to talk about on slips of paper. Collect the slips and discuss as a group the statements suggested.)

Option 2: Tally the group's responses. First collect the papers and redistribute them. Then read the first statement and ask the kids to raise their hands if the paper they received is marked "Agree." Now have them raise their hands if the first statement is marked "Disagree." Write the two totals on the board and ask for comments. Continue in the same way with as many of the statements as time allows.

Thinking Starters

Hand out copies of the "Factsheet on Abstinence" on page 102 and have a volunteer read the first section aloud. Ask if anyone was surprised by those facts. Ask different volunteers to read the other sections and discuss them as a group. Point out that these facts weren't written by a group of ministers—they were gathered by Planned Parenthood.

Ask why they think many couples are still not abstaining, in spite of these facts.

Discussion Starters

Pass out copies of "Secret Birth Control" on page 103. Divide into groups and have each group read the story and rank the characters. Afterward, have each group report its rankings. (Be careful not to get sidetracked into a discussion on abortion.)

Then ask:
• Which person in the story exhibited values most contradictory to Christian values?
• If you didn't have to worry about pregnancy or sexually transmitted diseases, would you have a different view of sex before marriage?

Faith Starters

Pass out copies of the "10 Principles of Sexual Behavior" on page 104. Have the group read each principle and the Scripture verses that go with it and think of one sentence that expresses the principle in a practical way. (Example for Principle Three, "Sexual behavior should honor God": I won't do anything sexually that would embarrass me in front of God.)

Action Starters

Pass out the "My Personal Sexual Standard" sheet on page 105 and have each person fill one out. Tell them to make it specific to cover any situation where sex may be involved.

Afterward, point out some practical ways to help keep a high standard:
• Inform any person you date that you do have high standards.
• Explain that if he or she pressures you sexually, the relationship is over.
• Don't allow yourself to get into a compromising situation.
• Don't act one way when you're in public and then suddenly have high standards on a date.
• Talk to an adult you trust if things are not going well.

Reflection Starters

Give everyone a copy of "Reflection Starters" on page 106 (or write one or more of the sentence stems on the board) and ask the students to complete the sentences. If you wish, collect the papers.

Session Nine: How Far Should You Go?

Prime-time TV has become a prime example of going all the way, all the time, with anyone, anywhere. At the same time, our sons and daughters are in the "prime" of their lives, faced with decisions concerning their own sexuality. They need to decide how they will respond now, before they are in a situation requiring an immediate decision (like the back seat of a car).

Why not open this discussion by talking about who set the standards for you when you dated? Again it's important not to force your opinion on your son or daughter, but to share your views and listen to his or hers.

In addition to discussing the questions below, as you watch TV together, try to think of some alternatives for characters who find themselves in sexually compromising situations.

Discussion Questions

For parents:
1. How far do you believe an unmarried couple should go?

2. Who set the standard when you were dating?

3. Were you a Christian when you were dating? Did it help?

For the son or daughter:
1. How far do *you* believe you should go?

2. Who do you believe should set the standard?

3. Do you believe God can help you hold to your standards?

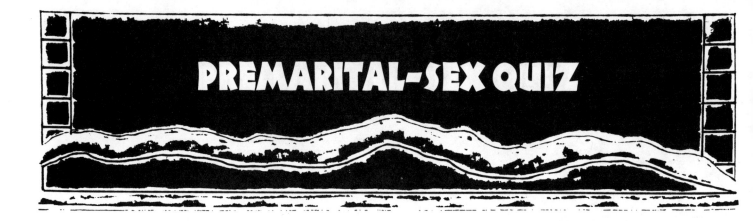

PREMARITAL-SEX QUIZ

Agree   Disagree   1. Being in love justifies premarital sex.

Agree   Disagree   2. If you're not ready for marriage, you're not ready for premarital sex.

Agree   Disagree   3. Promiscuity is a sin.

Agree   Disagree   4. Once you start having premarital sex, you might as well continue.

Agree   Disagree   5. Premarital sex bases a relationship on physical aspects.

Agree   Disagree   6. Everyone is doing it. It's natural.

Agree   Disagree   7. Having premarital sex helps a couple determine whether they are sexually compatible.

Agree   Disagree   8. Premarital sex must be wrong because couples have to sneak to do it.

Agree   Disagree   9. Many couples who have premarital sex feel guilty.

Agree   Disagree   10. The side effects of premarital sex include jealousy, possessiveness, guilt, and depression.

Agree   Disagree   11. Premarital sex offers a false sense of intimacy.

Agree   Disagree   12. People who have premarital sex are likely to cheat on their spouses after they are married.

Agree   Disagree   13. Love needs to be expressed through sex.

Agree   Disagree   14. Waiting is worth it.

Agree   Disagree   15. Having premarital sex will affect your reputation.

Agree   Disagree   16. If more people had premarital sex, there would be less pornography, prostitution, and perversion.

Agree   Disagree   17. Having premarital sex with one partner makes it easier to do it with others.

Agree   Disagree   18. Premarital sex makes a person feel wanted, cared about, and appreciated.

Agree   Disagree   19. God's laws are absolute regarding premarital sex. This makes it wrong no matter what the circumstances.

Agree   Disagree   20. Premarital sex provides people with a needed sexual release.

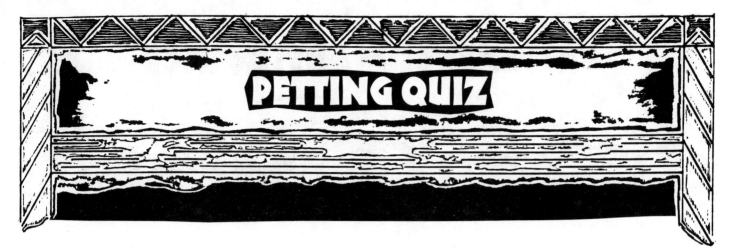

PETTING QUIZ

Agree   Disagree   1. Petting is permissible as long as you don't go all the way.

Agree   Disagree   2. Once you start petting, it's harder to say "no" to intercourse.

Agree   Disagree   3. Petting, for the most part, is a harmless activity.

Agree   Disagree   4. The Bible says nothing about petting, so why not?

Agree   Disagree   5. It feels good, so why not?

Agree   Disagree   6. Petting is permissible because it allows a couple to have sexual release without intercourse.

Agree   Disagree   7. Everyone is doing it. It's normal.

Agree   Disagree   8. Petting is an important learning experience for young people.

Agree   Disagree   9. Petting is as much a sin as sexual intercourse.

Agree   Disagree   10. If two people love each other, petting is permissible.

Agree   Disagree   11. Petting makes some people feel used and cheap.

Agree   Disagree   12. If you aren't ready for marriage, you aren't ready for petting.

Agree   Disagree   13. Petting bases a relationship on only physical aspects and neglects the spiritual ones.

Agree   Disagree   14. Petting with one partner makes it easier to do it with others.

Agree   Disagree   15. Petting is a good way to show your partner love and affection.

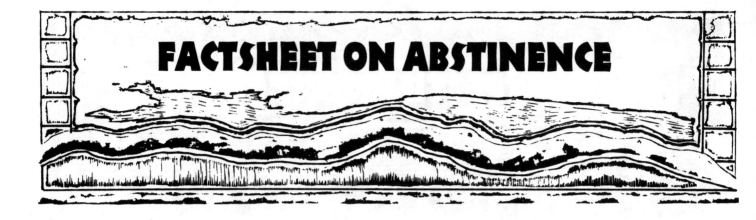

FACTSHEET ON ABSTINENCE

Facts

The majority of teens in the United States practice abstinence.

• 57% of males and 69% of females under 17 have never had intercourse. (Haas)

• 6 out of 10 males and 8 out of 10 females under age 16 have never had intercourse. (Norman)

• 40% of women polled wish they had delayed having sexual intercourse. 14% of men feel the same. (Sorenson)

Good Reasons to Choose Abstinence
Medical Reasons

• Abstinence is the only method of birth control that is 100% free of side effects.

• Abstinence reduces the risk of unwanted pregnancy. (Pregnancy can still occur if sperm is ejaculated near the entrance to the vagina during heavy petting.)

• Abstinence reduces the risk of contracting herpes, gonorrhea, and other sexually transmissible diseases. (STDs can still be passed by an infected person through contact with any mucous membranes or saliva.)

• Abstinence reduces the risk of cervical cancer. Cancer researchers are now suggesting a connection between early sexual activity, multiple sexual partners, and increased incidence of cervical cancer in women under 25.

Relationship Reasons

• A couple may find that delaying sexual intercourse contributes in a positive way to their relationship.

• Abstaining may allow a couple time to develop a deeper friendship. They may spend more time talking, building mutual interests, sharing their good times with other friends, and establishing an intimacy that is other than sexual.

• Abstaining can be a test of love. Counter to the old line "you would if you loved me," abstinence can allow time to test the endurance of love beyond the first attraction and before having sexual intercourse.

• Abstaining may contribute to teaching people to be better lovers, to explore a wide range of ways to express love and sexual feelings.

Personal Reasons

• Abstinence can be a sign of real emotional maturity and integrity. Many young women and men report feeling pressured into having sexual intercourse before they are ready. It requires maturity and honesty to be able to resist the pressure of someone you love in order to make a decision that is consistent with personal values and needs.

References

Haas, Aaron. *Teenage Sexuality*. New York: Macmillan, 1979.

Norman, Jane and Myron Harris. *The Private Life of the American Teenager*. New York: Rawson, Wade, 1981.

Sorenson, Robert. *Adolescent Sexuality in Contemporary America*. New York: World, 1973.

Adapted from material prepared by Planned Parenthood of Santa Cruz County, CA

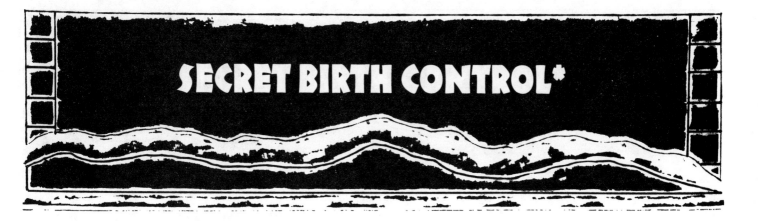

SECRET BIRTH CONTROL*

Robin didn't sleep around. She did sleep with her boyfriend, but that wasn't "sleeping around." She really loved Seth. She hoped someday they would get married. Sure, he wasn't the only boyfriend she had slept with, but people who love each other should have sex together. Sex is part of love.

Robin was eighteen and a senior—old enough to make her own decisions. She had always tried to be honest with her parents, but that didn't mean she told them everything. Now that she was eighteen, she decided to have a frank discussion with her parents (well, her mom anyway). She told her mom she thought it was okay to have sex with someone you love and, in fact, she had been having sex with Seth. She also told her mother she thought abortion was wrong and therefore wanted to use birth control.

Her mother was appalled at the whole conversation and refused to even discuss the possibility of birth control. She ordered Robin to break up with Seth and not have sex with anyone. Robin reminded her mother that she could order birth control pills without her permission. Her mother threatened to destroy any birth control pills or devices she found.

Robin continued having sex with Seth and acquired birth control pills through a local clinic. A couple of months later her mother found the pills and threw them away. Robin was so angry that she continued to have sex with Seth without any protection. Two months later she was pregnant. Since she didn't believe in abortion, she told Seth she was pregnant, fully expecting him to agree to get married. After all, they had been talking about it. She was shocked to discover that he had no intention of getting married and blamed her for getting pregnant in the first place.

"If you had used birth control pills, we wouldn't be in this mess," he told her.

"Well, what about you!" she yelled. "Why didn't you use protection?"

Seth replied sarcastically, "Because I'm not the one who can get pregnant!"

Robin broke up with Seth and had an abortion. All her parents knew was that she had broken up with Seth. They were very glad she had done as they had asked.

• Who was the most responsible for Robin's abortion?

• Rank the following characters from most responsible to least responsible:

_____ Robin

_____ Seth

_____ Robin's mom

Provide a reason for each ranking.

Scripture guide: Psalms 139:13-16; 1 Corinthians 6:13, 6:18-20; Proverbs 22:6; Ephesians 6:1-4

*Adapted with permission from *Amazing Tension Getters*, Zondervan/Youth Specialties, 1988.

10 PRINCIPLES OF SEXUAL BEHAVIOR

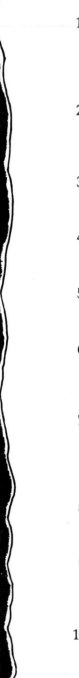

1. The Principle of Goodness
   Sex was created by God. Genesis 2:18-24
   There was no shame. Genesis 2:25
   Sex is beautiful. Song of Solomon
   Principle: *Sex is good.*

2. The Principle of Design
   Sex was designed to culminate in intercourse.
   So anytime you start, that's where it wants to end up.
   Principle: *Sex is fulfilled only in intercourse.*

3. The Principle of Honor
   We are to honor God with our bodies. 1 Corinthians 6:20
   Principle: *Sexual behavior should honor God.*

4. The Principle of Oneness
   When you have sex, two become one. Genesis 2:24; Matthew 19:5; 1 Corinthians 6:16
   Principle: *You give up part of yourself in sexual intercourse.*

5. The Principle of Temptation
   Sexual temptation can be handled. 1 Corinthians 10:13
   Principle: *We can resist sexual temptation.*

6. The Principle of Lust
   The longer you fool with sex, the more dangerous it is. James 1:12-15; 1 Thessalonians 4:3-8
   Principle: *Sexual foreplay is dangerous.*

7. The Principle of Running
   Sometimes the only way to deal with sexual temptation is to run, break off the relationship, take a cold shower. Genesis 39:12
   Principle: *Sometimes the only way to deal with sexual temptation is to make a radical break.*

8. The Principle of Love
   Love should be the guideline for our sexual behavior. 1 Corinthians 13:1-13
   Principle: *Love expresses itself in waiting.*

9. The Principle of Self-Control
   If you don't control your body, it will control you. 1 Thessalonians 4:4; 1 Corinthians 6:12-14; 1 Corinthians 10:23-24
   Principle: *When sex controls you, you've gone too far.*

10. The Principle of Consequence
    Sex is not a neutral act. There are always consequences. Galatians 6:7-8; Romans 1:24-25
    Principle: *Sex always has consequences.*

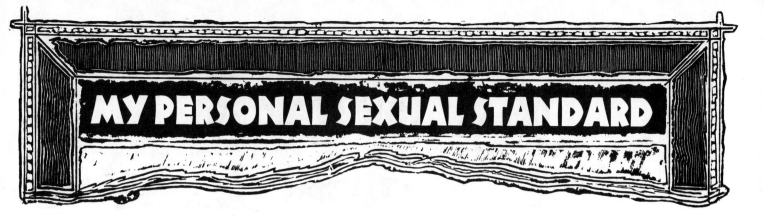

MY PERSONAL SEXUAL STANDARD

	I WILL	I WILL NOT
At school:		
The way I dress:		
With someone I like a little:		
On the phone:		
In a car:		
On a date:		
With someone I'm serious about:		
On the phone:		
In a car:		
On a date:		

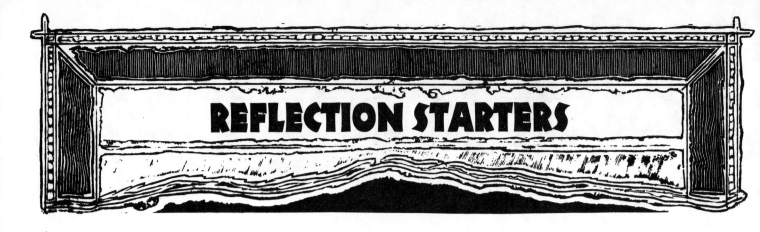

REFLECTION STARTERS

My sexual standard at this moment is:
   Non-existent   Not great   OK   Pretty good   Just right

I really need help in this area:

When it comes to my sexual standard and my relationship with God, I feel:

The best thing I learned from this session was:

SESSION TEN
THE OTHER CONSEQUENCES OF SEX

Session Purpose

To discuss the emotional, relational, and spiritual consequences of premarital sexual activity.

Background Brief

For a long time now the church has tried to discourage the sexual activity of its young by convincing them such behavior is contrary to the Bible. That's important, but it hasn't been very effective. Many adolescents believe that the only consequences of their sexual behavior will be pregnancy, STD, and the disapproval of God.

As a result, they are ignorant of the most common consequences of sexual activity— depression, guilt, and so on. Adolescents need to understand that sex is not just a physical act with physical consequences; it always has emotional, spiritual, and relational consequences as well.

Group Starters

This activity is simple but graphic. Squeeze the contents of a tube of toothpaste on a table. Tell the group you will give a volunteer $5 if he or she can get the toothpaste back in the tube. Invite someone to try.

After a few minutes, stop the volunteer and ask another person to come up. This time give him or her two pieces of paper that have been glued together. Again,

offer $5 if the volunteer can separate the papers without damaging either page. After a few minutes, point out that some things, once done, can't be undone. Ask what this has to do with sexual behavior.

Thinking Starters

Read Gary's story to the group and ask them to name the feelings he was experiencing. The list could include guilt, anxiety, suspicion, jealousy, depression, withdrawal, isolation, anger, insecurity, and low self-esteem.

Then read Linda's story and ask the group to name some of her feelings. Point out that in both cases those problems were the direct result of sexual involvement. Linda's sexual involvement was the single cause, and for Gary, it was one of the causes. Guide the group to see that sex has emotional (and for Linda, spiritual) consequences as well as physical ones.

Gary

Gary was still stunned. It had been a week and he was still walking around like a zombie. Cheri had broken up with him. How could she do that after ten months? Gary hated her. Then he loved her. Then he wished she was dead or hurt in a terrible car accident. He couldn't face anybody at school. They all knew. How could she do that? They had great sex and were going to get married in four years. While

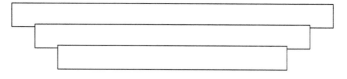

they went together, he'd given up his friends, let his grades drop, and quit sports . . . all for her. Gary felt so alone.

He wondered if Cheri had found someone else, someone like Don Henderson, Mr. Jock. He wanted to punch Henderson's lights out. But what good would it do? Gary knew he didn't have a chance against someone like that. He'd probably never get another girlfriend. He'd thought about quitting school or changing schools. He even considered suicide. Man, what's happening to me? he asked himself. I don't know what to do.

Linda
Linda walked in the door and ignored her parents. "Hi, honey," they said, "how was your date?" Linda ran into her room, flung herself on the bed, and began quietly crying. "Why did I let Bill do that?" she thought. They had parked after the game. They began kissing and the next thing she knew, he was unfastening her bra . . . and she let him and then his hands were all over her. She stopped him, but it was too late. How could she ever face him? How could she ever face her parents, her friends? What if he told his buddies?

Linda felt dirty and used, but most of all she knew she had let God down. She had wanted Bill to do what he did, yet she didn't want him to do it. She was so mixed up.

Discussion Starters

Give everyone a copy of "Consequences" on page 111 and ask each person to rank the items listed according to their importance in their decisions about premarital sex. Then divide the class into small groups and encourage (but don't insist) the kids to share how they ranked the items.

After the groups have had some time to talk it over, ask what they learned from this activity.

Faith Starters

Read the passage below to the group. Then ask them to listen as you read it again and stop you when they hear you describe a consequence of adultery. What are the implications of this passage for our own sexual behavior? Does the passage apply just to men lusting after women? Where does God fit into this? Can he rescue us from some of these complications? How?

Burnt Clothes and Scorched Feet

"For these commands are a lamp, this teaching is a light, and the corrections of discipline are the way to life, keeping you from the immoral woman, from the smooth tongue of the wayward wife. Do not lust in your heart after her beauty or let her captivate you with her eyes, for the prostitute reduces you to a loaf of bread, and the adulteress preys upon your very life.

"Can a man scoop fire into his lap without his clothes being burned? Can a man walk on hot coals without his feet being scorched?

"So is he who sleeps with another man's wife; no one who touches her will go unpunished. Men do not despise a thief if he steals to satisfy his hunger when he is starving. Yet if he is caught, he must pay sevenfold, though it costs him all the wealth of his house. But a man who commits adultery lacks judgment; whoever does so destroys himself. Blows and disgrace are his lot, and his shame will never be wiped away; for jealousy arouses a husband's fury, and he will show no mercy when he takes revenge. He will not accept any compensation; he will refuse the bribe, however great it is" Proverbs 6:23-35.

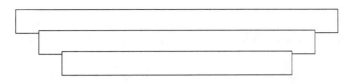

Action Starters

The Bible makes it clear that sex should wait until marriage. The question is, what should you do in the meantime?

Write the two questions below on the board and ask the young people to write themselves a letter, answering the questions. Have them put their letters in self-addressed envelopes and give them to you. Explain that you will mail them back to them in three to six months.

• What are you going to do as a result of this lesson? Why did you make those decisions? How are you going to make sure you stick to them?

• What can you do for friends who suffer or may suffer negative consequences of their sexual activity?

Reflection Starters

Write the question below on the board and ask everyone to think a moment before writing the answer. Collect the papers, if you wish.

What have you learned about sex and your relationship with God as a result of this session?

Session Ten: The Other Consequences of Sex

Much has been said about the "heavy" consequences of premarital sex, particularly pregnancy and sexually transmitted diseases. However, the more common consequences like guilt, jealousy, loss of self-respect, depression, insecurity, and anxiety go largely undiscussed. Young people need to realize that sexual activity outside of marriage has emotional and social consequences in addition to the physical ones.

To open this discussion with your son or daughter, talk about a friend (or even a relative, perhaps without identifying the person) who made sexual mistakes that led to consequences, ranging from an unwanted pregnancy to serious emotional distress. Or share something from your past that you wish you could do over, whether sexual or nonsexual. Stress that once some things are done, they can't be undone.

Discussion Questions

For parents:

1. Looking back on your high school years, do you have any regrets sexually?

2. What lessons did you learn from your mistakes that might help me now?

3. What do you think are the consequences of "fooling around"?

For the son or daughter:

1. What did you learn about the consequences of sex?

2. How can you avoid those consequences?

3. What can we do to help you?

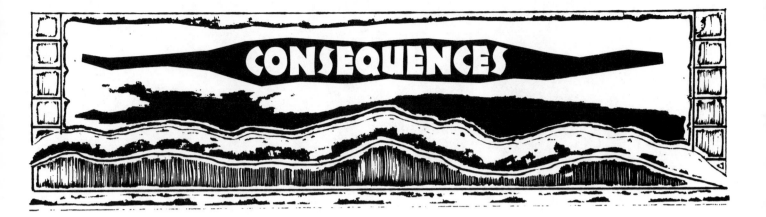

Rank each item below from 1 (most important) to 10 (least important) to show which consequences have the most influence on your decision concerning premarital sex.

_____ I fear pregnancy.

_____ I expect to feel guilty and lose self-respect.

_____ I fear my parents or other family members will find out.

_____ I worry about sexually transmitted diseases.

_____ I know it's against God's will.

_____ I have concluded that sex is overrated and may not be worth the risks.

_____ I worry that my partner will tell others.

_____ I want to enter marriage as a virgin.

_____ I worry that my partner doesn't really love me and will break up as soon as I "give in."

_____ I love my partner and desire to protect him or her from negative consequences of premarital sex.

SESSION ELEVEN
THREE PROBLEMS OF SEX

Session Purpose

To explore three of the many problems that increased sexual activity has caused in our society: sexually transmitted diseases (STDs), date rape, and sexual abuse.

Background Brief

According to the Center for Disease Control, the nation is in the grip of an STD epidemic that infects an average of 33,000 people a day. More and more cases are being reported among adolescents 15 and older. Of equal concern are the increasing reports of date rape and sexual abuse.

All three issues affect adolescents in and out of the church. Again, we continue to be haunted by the old myth that if you talk about certain subjects, you will make the problem worse. The truth is, talking about these issues helps those who for years have kept silent and have suffered greatly because of it.

Date rape is a new term for something that has been going on for a long time. Sexual abuse has also been around a long time, and finally the victims are gaining the courage to talk about it. It would be irresponsible not to cover these issues in a series on sex. Of course, there are many more topics, such as abortion and pornography, that we hope you will have an opportunity to cover in addition to the topics in this series.

Group Starters

Ask if anyone knows what STD means. If no one does, explain that it's short for sexually transmitted disease. Encourage the kids to name the STDs they know. Write the ones they name on the board. Then discuss each one, adding any in the list below that were not identified by the group.

AIDS

Acquired Immune Deficiency Syndrome, or AIDS, blocks the body's ability to fight off infection by destroying the immune system. Victims tend to die of pneumonia, cancer, and other problems brought on by their weak immune systems. Although scientists are working to develop a cure, they haven't found one yet. AIDS is transmitted by sexual contact that involves the exchange of body fluids, by blood-to-blood contact, by sharing contaminated needles, and from an infected mother to her unborn baby. It is NOT transmitted by hugging, touching, coughing, or eating or drinking after someone with AIDS.

Symptoms include a persistent fever, weight loss, swollen lymph glands, fatigue, and drenching night sweats. All of these symptoms, of course, can accompany other diseases, too. It may take three to eight years before the person develops these symptoms, which allows plenty of

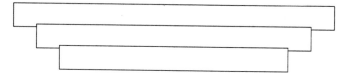

time for someone to spread AIDS without being aware of it.

Chlamydia

This disease infects three to ten million Americans a year. It is spread by sexual contact and by infected mothers during birth. For men, symptoms may be absent or include discharge from the penis or a burning sensation during urination. Women may have vaginal itching, chronic abdominal pain, or bleeding between menstrual periods. Four out of five women will notice nothing until complications set in, which include infertility (men and women) and pregnancy problems that can kill a fetus. There is a cure.

Genital Herpes

Twenty million Americans have genital herpes. Recurrences are frequent in some and rare in others. Some persons have only one outbreak in a lifetime. The symptoms include blisters in the genital area that turn into open sores. The initial outbreak is sometimes accompanied by swollen glands, headache, or fever. The lesions may last weeks. Later outbreaks are shorter and less severe. There is no cure.

Gonorrhea

The number of gonorrhea cases is on the rise after being stable for eleven years. Most infected women have no symptoms, but men show a pus-like discharge. The complications range from back pains and urination problems to arthritis and sterility. Babies of infected mothers may be born blind. There is an alarming increase in a strain of gonorrhea that resists the traditional cure of penicillin.

Syphilis

This disease is on the decline and is usually detected through a blood test. It has serious complications unless treated with penicillin.

Trichomoniasis

Men usually have no symptoms and women have a frothy discharge, itching, and redness of genitals. Complications include gland infections in women. There is a cure.

Venereal Warts

These warts can occur around the genitals or inside the cervix. Although they may be painless, they are dangerous, as babies exposed at childbirth may get warts in their throat. Some doctors believe these warts can increase the risk of cancer of the cervix, vulva, penis, and anus. They can be removed with a drug or surgery.

Explain that all of these diseases are transmitted almost exclusively by sexual intercourse or contact with the genital areas. That means you can get them *without* having intercourse. How do you keep from getting these diseases? It's very simple. Don't have sex. Don't fool around.

Thinking Starters

You might introduce the survey below by asking your young people for their own responses to each item and comparing their opinions to the results. Or, to save time, just read the results aloud.

This UCLA survey asked teenagers if it was all right if a male forced a female to have intercourse if:

	% Answering Yes Female	Male
He spent a lot of money on her?	12	39
She led him on?	27	54
They have dated a long time?	32	43
He was so turned on he thought he couldn't stop?	21	36
She said she was going to have sex with him and then changed her mind?	31	54
She let him touch her above the waist?	28	39
She was stoned or drunk?	18	39

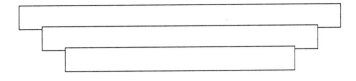

Ask the kids how they feel about the results. What do they tell us about the way most adolescents view date rape?

Have the group develop a definition of date rape. Do they think it's a problem in your community? Ask volunteers what they would do if sex were being forced on them. Would it make any difference who was doing it?

Discussion Starters

Pass out copies of one or both stories, "Stepfather Dilemma" on page 118 or "Big Date" on page 119. After discussing them as a class or in small groups, offer these suggestions for someone who is being sexually abused:

• Get professional help immediately. If you don't know anyone to go to, ask your youth worker or minister.
• Don't try to please everyone. It can't be done. You must save yourself from emotional and spiritual destruction. No one deserves being abused. If your parent or parents refuse to admit there is a problem, go to someone else.
• If you report abuse, chances are the offending person will end up in jail. Remember, it is not *your* fault. It is the other person's.
Note: If a young person tells you he or she has been abused, in many states you are required to report it to the local children's protective agency. Be sure to ask your pastor or minister about this issue if the need arises.

Faith Starters

The Bible doesn't say much about STDs, date rape, or sexual abuse. It does, however, offer a blueprint for spiritual and emotional healing:
Confront the issue head on. Sometimes in the church we "spiritualize" our problems: we put them in God's hands and ask him to take care of them. If you were raped, however, God will not report the rapist. You must do it. If you were abused, God will not expose the perpetrator. You must. Loving God does not mean we allow people to get away with sin and figure God will take care of them later. He doesn't want us to allow someone to destroy others when we could stop that from happening. At the same time, if you have contracted an STD, you need to face the problem, get medical help, and notify everyone you have had contact with.
Get help from God and others. Besides asking God for help, we must also seek help from those who have wisdom and experience. Most of the New Testament is composed of letters from church leaders giving advice and help in response to a call from others. Being a Christian means we understand that God has gifted certain people to help others in need.
Let God heal your emotions. These kinds of experiences can easily lead to bitterness and resentment. You will never get over the scars until your memories are healed and you are freed from the anger and resentment that enslaves you. Asking God to free you from anger doesn't negate the wrong that was done to you; instead, it frees you from the destructive consequences of that wrong.
Look forward, not back. The Christian view of hope is not just that someday we will be with God. The Christian view of hope means that we live each day looking forward, that we are free.

Optional: If you wish, close the meeting by reading "The Other Door" on page 120. Point out that Jesus can heal even the most horrible experiences. Ask if the group would like to talk further about how Christ can free them from their past and heal the memories.

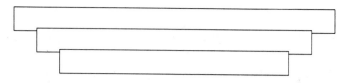

Action Starters

Divide into three small groups and have them each create a flyer for adolescents. One will be titled "How to Prevent Sexually Transmitted Diseases," one "What to Do If You Are Date Raped," and the third, "What to Do If You Are Sexually Abused." Make copies and encourage the kids to ask for permission to post the flyers at their schools and other appropriate places. Ask them to take the flyers home and discuss them with their parents.

Reflection Starters

Write the three questions below on the board. Read each aloud and allow two minutes of silence as the kids think about their answers to the questions. If you wish, encourage volunteers to share what they are thinking.
• Was this a difficult lesson for you? Why or why not?
• What was the most important thing you learned?
• What would you tell someone who was hurting from one of these experiences to comfort them and give them hope?

♂ PARENT DISCUSSION GUIDE ♀

Session Eleven: Three Problems of Sex

Tragically, date rape (forcing someone you know to have sex with you), sexually transmitted diseases, and sexual abuse are on the rise in this country. The nation is becoming increasingly aware of these issues, yet young victims still often live in fear and mistrust.

We need to care enough to learn more about these issues and communicate our concern to our children. Please take a few minutes to look over the flyers your son or daughter has brought home and discuss them.

Discussion Questions

For parents:
1. What would you add to the flyers?

2. How do you feel about these three areas?

For the son or daughter:
1. Have you ever had to deal with any of these problems?

2. How do you think we (your parents) would handle knowing you experienced any of these problems?

STEPFATHER DILEMMA

Denise has decided to run away. Her home life is horrible, and it's getting worse. She hates her stepfather. Actually, she's afraid of him. More than once he has made sexual advances toward her. Denise is afraid to tell anyone. Even if her mother did believe her, it could lead to another divorce. One divorce is enough for anyone to experience. Denise doesn't want anyone else to know either—not even Kevin, her boyfriend. She worries that maybe it's her fault her stepfather acts the way he does. Denise asks Kevin to loan her some money so she can go live with her father in another state.

- What would you do if you were Denise? Why?

- What would you do if you were Kevin? Why?

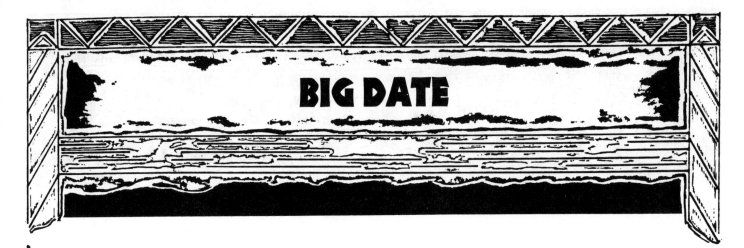

BIG DATE

Julie couldn't stop crying. In one night her fourteen-year-old life had completely come apart. She remembered being so excited when Mike asked her out. Her parents weren't so excited and didn't want to let her go at first. She had been really relieved when they finally said "yes."

She and Mike had gone to a party with some of his friends, but after an hour or so, he wanted to leave. Julie had been having a great time, but if Mike wanted to leave, that was all right with her.

He told her they would go get a hamburger, but when he parked on a dark road with no houses in sight, she found out her parents had been right about him after all. He kissed her a few times and then it was over almost before she knew what was happening. She still had a bruise on her chest where he had held her down on the seat with his elbow. She couldn't even think about the rest of it. She just knew she wasn't a virgin anymore, and she hadn't even had a choice.

I might be pregnant, she worried over and over. Or maybe he has some kind of disease and now I have it. What am I going to do?

• What advice could you give Julie?

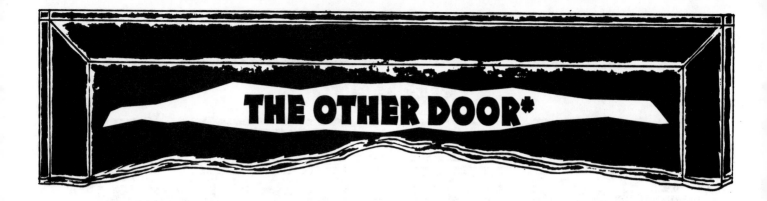

THE OTHER DOOR*

I'm a nineteen-year-old girl. Eight years ago, my uncle, who was in his 40s at the time, began coming into my bedroom late at night. He wanted to have sex. I was only eleven! The first couple of times, I tried to fight him, but after that I just gave in and let him have his way. Somehow I believed I had seduced him and it was my fault.

This went on for two full years, and then he moved away. By that time it was too late for me. I've had sex since then with any guy who wanted to, and I've been called every name in the book for "easy."

Besides all that, I've become hopelessly addicted to crack. I'm sure you can't help, Mr. Wilkerson, but I had to tell somebody.

Mr. Wilkerson, I'm writing to tell you about the unbelievable victory that is happening in my life. The night I walked out of the office where you and the other ministers prayed for me, I never dreamed I would face the devil's attack as soon as I did.

I met my girlfriends in the parking lot, and we got in the car for the five-hour ride back to the university. Sitting in the back seat, I laid my head back. I hoped to sleep the entire trip home.

We hadn't been driving for five minutes when all of a sudden I felt the car fill up with the presence of Satan. Having felt this many times before, I knew at that moment I was about to face my first great battle as a new Christian.

All of a sudden, I had a vision. It was so clear I felt like I was looking at a television set. The scene was a flashback to my old bedroom, and I was sitting on the bed as an eleven-year-old. I saw my uncle open the door and walk in like he did the first time it ever happened.

My uncle reached out his arms and beckoned me to come to him. I had learned that those arms were very cruel. In that moment, sitting in that car, I knew that if I yielded to my uncle's wishes, I would remain the same.

The battle was on as we traveled at 60 miles per hour. The other girls had no idea that the devil was trying to snuff out the work Jesus had done in my life that night.

As the vision continued, my uncle insisted that I come to him. Mr. Wilkerson, I was about to enter my uncle's arms as tears of pain poured down my cheeks. But then, hearing the door latch turn, I saw the door open a second time.

To my amazement, standing in the doorway with tears streaming down his face was Jesus! He reached his nail-scarred hands in my direction and said, "Come unto me."

For the first time in my life, I realized that I had another door available to me. Turning away from my uncle, I raced into the loving arms of my big brother Jesus.

Instantly, the vision was over, and I was weeping. My girlfriends asked me what was wrong. For the rest of the drive home I wept and repeated over and over again, "I'm free . . . I'm free . . . I'm free. . . ."

* Reprinted with permission from *Straight Answers To Tough Questions About Sex* by Rich Wilkerson. Whitaker House: Springdale, PA, 1987.

SESSION TWELVE
THE PARDONABLE SINS

Session Purpose

To proclaim the good news about sexual sin—that no matter what you've done or what's been done to you, it *can* be forgiven.

Background Brief

The message too often given to adolescents is that sexual sins are *un*pardonable; they are the worst sins. It is easy for some adolescents, after a series of lessons about sex, to feel worse than they did before the course. Once young people hear God's high standards for sexual conduct, some feel it's too late and there's no hope. They need to realize that forgiveness isn't easy, but it's available to anyone and everyone.

Another problem, ironically, is that adolescents sometimes don't take forgiveness seriously enough. The "it's no big deal" syndrome takes over and forgiveness just becomes something you sprinkle on your past and move on. Forgiveness is free . . . but it's also hard. This session will deal with both aspects.

Group Starters

Begin by asking the group to brainstorm everything they know about God's forgiveness. Write their responses on chart paper or newsprint without evaluating their "correctness."

Then read aloud Luke 7:36-50 and John 8:1-11. Ask the group to list everything those passages say about forgiveness. (For example: look for insights from the past, made whole in the sight of God, cleansed, past forgiven and forgotten, no condemnation, free to go on, admission of sin, gratefulness, peace, etc.) Is there anything else they could add to their "word map" for forgiveness?

Thinking Starters

Read one or more of the three "Letters" on page 124 aloud and ask the group to respond. Or divide into three groups and have each group respond to a different letter and share its response with the larger group. What, if any, information from the Scripture they just read applies to these situations?

Discussion Starters

Have the group list every sexual sin they can think of, with several volunteers writing them on separate pieces of paper. Then point out that no matter what the sin, no matter how terrible the sin may be, it can be forgiven.

Ask the kids to crumple up the pieces of paper and throw them into a large empty coffee can. Now take a match and light the papers and let them burn completely out. Notice how much ash is left. It represents the consequences, the scars, the remains of sin. Sin always has consequences that live on even after forgiveness.

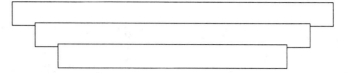

Talk about the woman caught in adultery in John 8. What happened to her afterward? What scars did she have to deal with? What remains were left for her?

Faith Starters

Have the kids read these Bible passages: Isaiah 38:17; 43:25; Psalm 103:11-12; and Micah 7:18-19. Ask them to notice all the word pictures used to describe sin and forgiveness.

Then have each person (or small group) choose the passage which is most meaningful to them. Give them some art supplies, and have them create their own forgiveness word pictures. Encourage each person or group to share the meaning of the picture with the other young people.

Action Starters

Repeat the activity described under "Discussion Starters," but this time give each person a piece of magicians' flash paper. (You can purchase it at a novelty store. It comes in 8½" by 11" sheets that you can cut into 3" squares. Don't tell the kids what it is!) Ask everyone to write his or her own sexual sins on the paper. Assure them no one will see what they write.

Have everyone crumple up the paper and throw it in a large, empty coffee can. Stand back and throw a lighted match into the can, as before. **This time make absolutely sure no one is right next to the can or looking into it. Everyone should be at least four feet away!!!** The results will be quite spectacular. There will be a large flash as the papers explode.

Now, ask the kids to look in the can. They will be surprised to find that the can is completely empty. No ash. No residue. The papers have completely disappeared.

Point out that our personal sin is not only forgiven, it is forgotten. God will remember our sin no more. It's completely gone. Ask what that means. Does it mean that a person who has had sexual intercourse can ask for forgiveness, and be considered a virgin as far as God is concerned?

Reflection Starters

Give everyone a copy of "Reflection Starters" on page 125 (or write one or more of the sentence stems on the board). Have them complete the sentences, but do not collect the papers.

Session Twelve: The Pardonable Sins

The message too often given to adolescents is that sexual sins are unpardonable; they are the worst sins. In fact, some adolescents, after a series of lessons about sex, feel worse than when they started. After they hear God's high standards for sexual conduct, they think it's too late and there is no hope, even for their thoughts concerning sexuality.

In this lesson we've talked about the forgiveness that God offers us, extending even to sexual sins. Nevertheless, adolescents often feel they have failed their parents by sinning sexually. If you learned your son or daughter had been involved sexually and was trying to work out this complex problem, how forgiving could you be?

Think of ways you can encourage your child to come to you with any problems, including sexual ones. Work through the questions below together and ask your son or daughter to rate you on a 1-10 scale as to how available and encouraging you are. Then together work out some ways you can improve on your communication.

Discussion Questions

For parents:

1. I know God would forgive me for sexual sins, but would you, as my parents?

2. If I had really messed up sexually, could I come to you and get good advice, or would you totally freak out?

3. Did you ever mess up? How did you deal with the guilt and the consequences?

For the son or daughter:

1. If you had sinned sexually, who would you go to for help? Be honest!

2. What one thing would you be afraid to tell us?

3. Can we make a deal? You feel free to come to us with your sexual problems, and we'll promise not to freak out or lock you in your bedroom until you're 21.

LETTERS

I need help. I'm writing to you because I trust you. I have this problem with sexual thoughts. Every time I see a neat-looking girl, I think about having sex with her. I think about her undressed, etc. I know it's wrong and I keep asking for forgiveness, but the very next day my mind is going crazy again. What's wrong? If God forgives me, how come I still have the problem?
Dennis

Here's my problem. I like sex. I enjoy all the stuff that you do with someone of the opposite sex. I know a lot of it is wrong and I don't want God getting mad at me and dissolving my lips. I want God to forgive me, but I don't want to stop doing this stuff, either. I mean, can I just keep doing this stuff and asking him to forgive me, even though I know I'm going to do it again? I figure I can keep having sex and then ask him to forgive me because he has to, doesn't he?

Abby

Look, I might as well be honest. I haven't just sinned. When it comes to sex, I've SINNED! You don't want to know what I've done, with whom, and how many times. Take my word for it, I've been real bad. I've had VD. I've had an abortion. The whole bit. But I am sick of all that stuff. I want to change my life, but does God really forgive someone like me? Really? I'm having a hard time believing that. I'm used and damaged goods, if you know what I mean. Do you think God will really forgive me?
Lisa

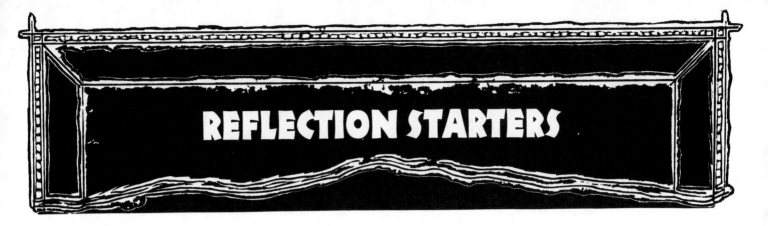

REFLECTION STARTERS

The hardest thing to believe about forgiveness is:

I believe God has forgiven me, but I'm not sure of:

I believe God forgives, but there is one thing I keep doing over and over again, and I wonder if God will keep forgiving me. That one thing is:

The most important thing I learned in this session was:

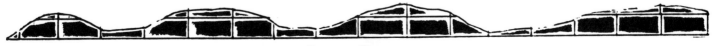